TO DEAR VERE
" ENJOY "

Robyn Elizabeth Welch

Exploring Dimensions
with the Body

A medical intuitive's
guide to natural healing

LOVING ENERGY

Robyn Welch

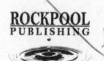

ROCKPOOL
PUBLISHING

A Rockpool book
Published by Rockpool Publishing
1/2 Cooper Street, Double Bay, NSW 2028, Australia
www.rockpoolpublishing.com.au

First published in 2008
Copyright © Robyn Elizabeth Welch, 2008

National Library of Australia Cataloguing-in-Publication Entry

Welch, Robyn Elizabeth.

Exploring dimensions with the body: the true sixth sense
story of a medical intuitive/Robyn Elizabeth Welch.

Welch, Robyn Elizabeth.
Healers — Biography.
Healing.

615.852092
Includes index

Typeset by Prototype Pty Ltd, Sydney, Australia
Printed and bound by Griffin Press, Adelaide, Australia

10 9 8 7 6 5 4 3 2 1

TABLE OF CONTENTS

SECTION ONE
My Healing Techniques Evolve

1 Born to Heal   2
2 Mother Nature's University   22
3 Bodies Reveal Their Secrets   42
4 Fly to Emotional Freedom   68

SECTION TWO
New Dimensions in Healing

5 London for the Twenty-First Century   91
6 The Human Energy Field   105
7 Embryos from the Heart   122
8 Frequency Wars   140
9 Electronic Bugs   164

SECTION THREE
Progress on the Pacific Coast

10 Animals Also Evolve   180
11 Suddenly, Vancouver   205
12 Accessing Higher Dimensions   223
13 My ER   252
14 Into a Healthy Twenty-First Century   267

FOREWORD

With the increasing understanding and awareness of quantum physics, we can be confident that these principles extend to every aspect of life.

Robyn Welch is at the forefront of applying these principles to health and illness.

I have been associated with Robyn for a decade, and have observed her work first hand.

I have no hesitation in recommending this book – a compelling account of her work and experiences in this realm of healing.

– Dr John A Walck MD, Seattle, USA

The use of energy and vibrations for healing is a fascinating subject. Ancient knowledge describes the interconnected webs of energy that bind the universe. Now the observations from quantum physics are discovering how true these teachings really are.

In the quantum world, the strange behaviours of atoms, subatomic particles, light and energy are observed. Einstein was the first to demonstrate that energy and matter are essentially the same. Even more amazing was the discovery that entangled particles can communicate and affect each other instantaneously, even if they have been separated to opposite ends of the universe. Particles flip in and out of existence as they move between matter and anti-matter. The rules that seem to work in everyday life, do not apply to the quantum world.

Robyn describes her work as the place where quantum physics and spirituality meet. Eventually we may understand exactly how such healing might work.

The story of Robyn's life is truly amazing. I am intrigued by Robyn's work as a diagnostician and healer. Robyn's clients are testimony to her ability to harness and support the power of innate self-healing that resides in each of us.

The challenge for modern medicine is to systematically investigate the work of Robyn and others like her to improve our understanding of health and wellbeing. Matter and energy are interchangeable. This knowledge provides us with infinite possibilities for healing and transformation.

– Dr Jennifer Hunter, Australia

My Healing Techniques Evolve

"...each one of us has within himself a deeper nature, and, of course, this deeper nature, being an eternal unity with God, or with the Living Spirit, is more than man; it is where the being of man, or the nature of man, merges into the Being of God..."

Ernest G. Holmes
Science of Mind

Chapter One

Born to Heal

"Go ahead, plunge right in. You can do it Robyn. Don't be afraid."

Quaking with fear, I took a deep breath, curled my small hands into fists, as my father had shown me, and dove headfirst into the river sixty feet below, wind whooshing past me at alarming speed. I plummeted to the bottom of the murky water, terrified that my lungs would explode and I'd never see daylight again. When at last I burst through the surface and heard my father shouting his approval, I knew that I could do anything I set my mind to. I was twelve years old.

I've often reflected on this incident, recognising it as a signpost on my journey to becoming a diagnostic medical intuitive. Healing often requires plunging into unknown dimensions of life to help people and being fiercely determined to succeed in the face of obstacles. It also requires a spiritual connection to the One Source, which I became aware of over time. Spiritual healing is not a job for the fearful or the faint of heart.

Even before I was a year old, my dad was determined to shape me into a strong and courageous person. Some would say he was trying to compensate for the fact that my older brother had been born with Down's Syndrome and would never be a high achiever in any field. If Dennis couldn't do it, then by gum Robyn could.

Fortunately, I was up to most challenges. I was a high-spirited, adventurous child who enjoyed climbing trees, riding horses, and winning swimming medals in our sunny suburb of Sydney, Australia. There was more to my life than athletics, however. From the time I could toddle, my heart went out to injured or sick animals in our neighbourhood, and I brought them home to bind up bleeding paws, splint broken wings, and minister to their every need. I once led a horse that looked exhausted back to our yard, not in the least concerned that he was attached to the milkman's wagon. The neighbours generally agreed, "The little Welch girl has a way with animals" and brought me furred and feathered patients to mend.

Our tight-knit family provided me with love and security. We were an affectionate bunch, always hugging and kissing members of our extended family and friends. My mother was a beautiful lady who taught me manners and made sure I developed habits of cleanliness. When I was eleven, she wrote a speech for me to deliver on the occasion of my winning a major horse event and taught me to practice speaking to an audience. Her encouragement made me feel appreciated and special.

My father was polished and well dressed and always expected me to be the same. But more importantly, I was to be brave. "Go on, it won't hurt you," was a common phrase he instilled in me about so many things from swimming in freezing water at five a.m. to stuffing huge pills far down the throats of ailing horses. He taught me sportsmanship and how to stay on the positive side of virtually every situation.

My plucky grandmother walked three miles to our home every day to help my mother care for Dennis' special needs. Granny Penny knew how to treat every condition, from broken bones to pneumonia, with a good dose of castor oil first on her list of remedies. She was generous to a fault. My uncle once commented that we should not give her valuable gifts for her birthday, as she'd just give them away to someone "more deserving."

Granny Penny's wisdom included a deep understanding of spirituality. Her very presence filled our lives with a profound sense of goodness and love. She taught me about God and though she was not a churchgoer, she saw to it that I went to the nearby Anglican Church and Sunday School where they taught me about Jesus. I learned that God is Love and still believe it, though not in the exact form that the ministers taught us.

A dark cloud fell over my carefree childhood when my lovely mother died of cancer. My heart felt as though it had broken in two. Not only was I totally bereft, but at the age of 13, I had to shoulder a huge amount of responsibility for keeping the house clean, making meals, and caring for Dennis and Bronwyn, my little sister. I had always taken it upon myself to protect my brother from nasty comments from people who didn't understand Down's Syndrome, but now his day-to-day needs became my responsibility.

Granny Penny still came to help out and between the two of us, we kept life on reasonably even keel for fifteen months. Then suddenly she was felled by a heart attack. With both my beloved mother and grandmother gone, my sorrow seemed a bottomless pit. Though I was winning riding competitions and was on track to go to university, I had to give it all up when the entire burden of housework and childcare fell on me. My father, formerly so encouraging, had been overwhelmed by my mother's death and no longer took a positive view of life. He declared that girls didn't need university degrees and that was that.

I've wondered whether I might have tried for medical school if I'd been able to continue my studies. But I have no regrets. Today, I believe that it was my destiny from the start to develop a new way of healing, something I might never have considered had I become a physician. However, my father told me that he'd pay for medical school for my son if he wanted to attend, so perhaps his intention provided some impetus for me to become a healer.

Try as I might, I couldn't keep up with the mountain of

chores each day brought. At the age of 16, heartbroken, unhappy, and with my confidence shattered, I had what the doctor termed a "nervous breakdown." He suggested that I get a job outside the home, which I took with relish, first working in a jewelry shop and then, when I was 18, taking a commuter train daily to Sydney where I worked as a junior designer in a furniture store. There I gloried in working with fine fabrics, combining colours and textures to create beautiful harmony. I felt closer to my mother while working as a designer, as she had been the one to teach me a love of fashion.

At about this time, my father sent Dennis to a "facility," as he had not fared well since my mother and Granny Penny died. When I went to see him, he wouldn't even talk to me. I was deeply saddened, knowing that I had lost my brother for all time.

I did keep up with my riding and swimming, continuing to win awards. The horses in my life taught me love and nurturing and I also learned a lot about physiology by caring for them. Most of all, I learned to communicate clearly, as horses cannot respond to vague directions. My athletic ability has helped me to overcome emotional and physical problems all my life. I believe that part of the reason I can do energy healing is that I keep myself in superb physical shape. It's as though I'm providing a healing blueprint for those whose bodies are weak and failing.

By the time I was 18, I was going out on casual dates

with several young men, two of whom proposed. My father approved of Max, a handsome seafaring Australian who looked smashing in uniform. The fact that he drank too much set off my alarm bells, but I was too smitten to listen to them. We had a glorious wedding in St. Andrew's Cathedral in Sydney and settled into an apartment in Cronulla, a sun-filled suburb right on the beach. Six months later, I became pregnant.

After daylong labour pains, my first thought as they handed my beautiful little Jane to me in the delivery room was, "I would give my life for this child." I'd never felt love so powerful before. For me, as for many other women, giving birth was a true spiritual experience. And when they wheeled me down the hall to my room at three in the morning, the walls literally began to glow with what I knew to be God's presence. I thought this glow was a natural part of childbirth and was surprised to learn that my girlfriends had not experienced similar manifestations of spirit.

Childbirth brings forth a very high level of energy. Sadly, some women cannot handle the vibrational lift and sink into post-partum depression. There's a kind of mental, physical, spiritual and emotional fitness that can be taught to expectant mothers to improve the quality of the experience for them and for their babies.

Jane's birth heralded a happy and active period. I designed special outfits for her and found it so enjoyable,

I began making clothing for Max and myself. I saw the opportunity to become a professional designer and branched out into creating a line of clothing to sell at children's boutiques.

I wanted more children as soon as possible. Sarah was born two years after Jane and Aaron followed two years later. I went back to riding in a big way, winning medals at arenas all over the area. I purchased an ailing horse that I nursed back to health and turned into a fine racehorse, in the process acquiring a reputation as a "horse whisperer." People from all over Australia brought their horses to me. As I trained them, I became aware that some horses had the uncanny ability to read my mind, responding to the idea of a command before I ever spoke it aloud. I worked to establish this extrasensory connection with horses, honing my ability to communicate with them at a subtle level. I had no idea at the time that this ability would one day evolve into talking to human organs and restoring them to health.

During this expansive period of happy family life, my intuition was growing too. It manifested in many small ways including giving friends spontaneous psychic readings without really intending to do so. Bewildered, I sought out books and classes that would help explain my unusual abilities. Back then, very little was available in Australia, where the search for answers to spiritual phenomena had barely begun. I managed to find *The Third Eye* by

T. Lobsang Rampa, a man who claimed to have been raised in a Tibetan lamaserie. Though some critics believed he'd never set foot in Tibet, the author had at least done his homework and I learned valuable lessons about tapping into universal energy and using the power to help others and ourselves. It made perfect sense to me.

Sadly, our idyllic family life was not to last. Max suffered business reversals, spiraled down into depression and became a problem drinker. We lost our lovely home and savings and lived at the edge of poverty. I helped out by giving riding lessons and even mucking out stables — anything to keep my children clothed and fed.

Our difficult situation turned into a full-fledged crisis in 1979 when I was diagnosed with a uterine tumour. I was terrified that I would die early, as my mother had, and leave my children to get along without me. I couldn't bear the thought.

A few nights before surgery was scheduled, an astonishing notion liberated my mind from worry and fear. It seemed to come from nowhere and everywhere: I would heal myself. The idea seemed unbelievable at first, but I quickly banished all negative thoughts and accepted it. At the deepest level of my being, certainty took root. I didn't hear voices or see visions; I just knew that I should bring white light through the energy centre in the centre of my forehead and guide it through my body to the tumour. T. Lobsang Rampa had written about this "third eye"

9

region, claiming it was a highly charged energy centre.

I went to work, willing light to enter and accumulate until I felt my forehead pulsating with energy. I made a great effort to increase this pure energy until enough accumulated to direct it in a fine ray through my body to my lower abdomen. Concentrating harder than I had ever done before, I sent the ray into the tumour, intending that it destroy it. I repeated this process the next day. When I reported to the hospital for surgery, the doctor could find no evidence that the tumour had ever been there.

"I zapped it with my energy ray," I said, delighted to have incontrovertible evidence that I'd developed an effective self-healing method.

His condescending reaction let me know that it was not safe to discuss energy healing with physicians, at least not back then. Now some are acquainted with and respectful of what they term "alternative" healing methods. In my opinion, energy healing is the natural way to heal a great many conditions; conventional medicine seems more like an alternative to me.

After I destroyed my tumour, my psychic awareness increased rapidly. I became more sensitive to vibrations of lingering past events and found myself intuitively picking up details of people's lives. As my sixth-sense abilities increased, I worked at keeping myself centred and grounded. I knew that I was developing something very special. Where it would all lead, I couldn't be sure, but

I knew it was important to keep on. Over and over, the word "purity" came into my mind and I knew that wherever I was going, it was pure. Pure energy? Pure light? I had no way to know as yet.

And then disaster struck. Driving home with three friends after a girls' night out, I was in a terrible auto accident. Passing drivers helped my three friends out of the wreckage but left me for dead in the back seat, as they could find no pulse. When paramedics arrived thirty minutes later, they discovered a weak pulse and carefully pried me from the ruined car. I had severe head injuries and a broken arm and collarbone. My right foot was almost severed and my spine was fractured in three places. My speech was slurred, my mind befuddled, I experienced double vision, and all of my other senses were diminished. Over the course of subsequent decades, three top clairvoyants, who knew nothing of my history, said I died in a car and was physically reborn, although I have no memory of "crossing over".

It would be nine years before I could function with a reliable degree of wellness. During that interminable time, Max was no help to me at all and physicians could do little. I vowed to go it alone with God's help. Inspired by my success of removing my tumour, I believed I could reprogram my mind and body — though I had sustained so much neurological damage I was incapable of using my energy ray. Day after day I struggled to think straight and speak correctly and to move through ordinary activities of life in spite of a pronounced weakness in my injured leg and a terrible limp. My physical pain never let up and I constantly fought off negative emotions of frustration and anger, common among persons with neurological impairment.

My children were wonderful to me, helping as much as they could, but the situation with Max deteriorated and in the midst of my battle to regain my health, Max and I were divorced. The bank took our property and I had to move my children into another house where I continued to work at healing myself.

As my self-healing practices grew stronger and my physical condition improved, I demonstrated a psychic reading technique using a flower on Sydney television and from that appearance came an invitation to become part of a large psychic fair. On the first day, I gave ordinary readings about people's lives and relationships, the information visible to me in their auras, or energy fields as we call them today. My clients were all reluctant to get out of their chairs afterward, lingering in silence. I was puzzled, knowing nothing of altered states, which I now realise they were experiencing. Halfway through the day, I was somehow moved to give advice about what vitamins or health treatments they needed. On the second day, I realised that I could see inside people's bodies, feeling their conditions with what I can only describe as deep knowing. I didn't try to heal them, but felt I could diagnose their conditions accurately. What was going on?

I began to wonder whether God wanted me to become a serious healer. Nothing would have made me happier, but one does not take on such an enormous responsibility lightly. I wasn't ready. If I were to help people regain their health, I'd need to learn anatomy, among other things. I was still devoting a considerable amount of energy to healing myself. A year went by before I made up my mind.

I formulated a prayer telling God that I wanted to diagnose correctly, to heal as well as Jesus did, and asking for a sign too strong to ignore. The sign was not long in coming, but for some reason, I took a different direction, perhaps just to get other aspirations out of my system.

My insurance case was finally settled, with the judge awarding me the maximum amount allowed under Australian law. It was 1988, and with all three of my children in college, I was free to create a new life.

I decided to set up a business in Manila to manufacture clothing. I was still not entirely well, but I thought I could make it work, travelling back and forth frequently. It was a great adventure for me, but between my lack of business experience and the political unrest in the Philippines, I suffered financial loss and emotional upheaval. I devised a different plan for my business in Manila, manufacturing only garments that I had presold to exclusive boutiques in Sydney. For a while, I enjoyed a degree of success, but when Australia suffered a recession in 1992, the market for expensive clothing dried up. I was disillusioned and tapped out. Worst of all, I had no love in my life. My children were far away and friends weren't calling.

To recover my energy and my joy in life, I jogged on the beach at Cronulla for miles each day, thrilled to feel my energy returning with every stride. I entered marathons with 46,000 other runners, amazing high-energy events. As I became progressively more physically fit, feelings of connectedness to God returned. I realised that I was in training not just for the races but also for the rest of my life.

I worked hard to raise my vibrational level and recovered my mental, spiritual, and emotional well being along with the physical. My foray into the fashion business had been instructive, but apparently was not my God-given purpose on this earth. Designing and sewing would be a way to make extra money in the future, not the main thrust of my life.

A series of delightful events occurred in Cronulla that underscored my growing belief that I had a higher path to follow. My friend Melissa noticed that my living room walls were glowing. I'd seen it too, but dismissed it as a trick of light. Other friends came to take a look and they determined that bright white light actually shone from the walls, its beams extending about six feet. Perhaps Divine energy was present because I'd worked so intensely in this room to raise my vibrational level, pulling myself out of negativity, worry, and despair. On another occasion, my cousin and I drove toward the end of a rainbow and actually caught up with it, a physical impossibility, I understand. We drove through a shower of brilliant colour for ten minutes. Twice after that, rainbows came right onto the balcony of my fifth floor apartment. And most delightful of all, while gazing at the sea at night, I saw myself sitting in the curve of the crescent moon as clearly as if I were watching a Technicolor movie.

A dozen times over the next year, I experienced terrifying surges of energy radiating through my head, producing the feeling that I was lifting off the ground. I felt this to be the merging of my earthly awareness with my spiritual being. It was a very powerful shift. I knew somehow that the two levels of consciousness must merge and strive for the energy needed to stay connected to the highest vibrational level available to human beings.

This is not an easy process. Many people get to this point in their spiritual development and pull back. However, those who can handle the powerful shift may go on to live in a high and happy state that allows them to accomplish meaningful spiritual work.

Next came an improbable but very important step in my journey. A man I barely knew invited me to Hawaii. Friends thought I was quite mad, but I trusted that all would be well. He had a condo with two bedrooms in lovely Kauai, one of the most beautiful islands in the world. I was spellbound with its magic. Four days into the trip, Ron was called home to Australia leaving me to enjoy Kauai on my own. Enchanted with its loveliness, I communed with the spirits of land, sea, and sky, engulfed with the most extraordinary positive energy I'd ever experienced anywhere.

I was invited to a New Year's Eve party at the magnificent Princeville Hotel to say hello to 1994. As the clock struck twelve, I took the hand of an older American woman named Alberta, intending to wish her happy New Year, but "Goodness, darling, you are having gallbladder trouble," popped out instead. It was an accurate diagnosis, and she called on me for four healing sessions before she left Hawaii. I was thrilled. I had wanted the power to diagnose and heal, and I was doing just that on this magical isle. Moreover, I'd taken a big stride into my new life. No turning back now.

Alberta went back to the mainland but friends of hers began to call me for healing sessions. Thank God I was not faced with anything too difficult and was able to help everyone who came to see me. Word spread quickly and my reputation grew. There was a steady stream of clients, some of them calling from the mainland to make appointments to fly to Kauai. As more people showed up with different ailments, my abilities seemed to keep pace with their needs.

During this time, I was seeing inside bodies more

clearly, viewing more of the organs needing the help that I was somehow able to provide. I had to learn to stay free from my clients' negative energy, which was thick in the fields of those who were ill. The worse their health, the more negative energy I had to fight through. I did this by producing forceful positive energy to counteract it. During this period, my energy became stronger and more powerful, enabling me to give several sessions every day.

One of the most interesting cases was Arthur, a man who had been injured in an accident years earlier and still suffered from lack of focus. I could see a pocket of fluid trapped in his brain and worked to remove it. When he came to see me the next day, the area was clean and his mind was clear. I was delighted, as I was all too familiar with frustrating problems brain injuries can inflict.

Though I was blossoming into a fully-fledged healer on Kauai, I did not feel right about taking money for my services. My financial situation was precarious so I turned once again to horses to earn my living expenses.

Then came a fateful call from one of my clients from California. She was so thrilled with the improved state of her health, she wanted me to come to San Francisco, where many of her friends would come for sessions and pay me for my services. Delighted, I set off with high expectations.

My son, Aaron, who was attending college in San Francisco, picked me up at the airport and took me to the affordable little hotel he'd booked for me. I told him about my work with some trepidation, wondering whether he would accuse me of being "woo-woo" or would be comfortable with his mum doing energy healing. I needn't have worried. His sensible response was to suggest that I ask clients for letters verifying that I'd helped them.

I remained in San Francisco for four months and the healing work went well. Invitations from other Americans took me to Florida for awhile, followed by a rather meandering trip with stops in Georgia, Alabama and Tennessee. Working with clients along the way, I realised that I no longer needed to concentrate on bringing the light into my forehead before directing it as a ray. Just one deep breath for centring and my energy ray was poised and ready.

At the end of 1994, I returned to Australia in time for Christmas with my children. Initially, I thought I'd stay, but natural healing was in its infancy in my homeland at that time, and I would need more people to work with to master my profession and prove this method. In America, significant numbers of people were open to and looking for healers. By March 1995, it became abundantly clear to me that I belonged in the USA where my work was appreciated, and back I went. It was the "path with a heart," as I loved my work and also loved the Americans whose hearts and minds were ready to participate in alternative healing. The genuine heart energy that emanates from most Americans is unparalleled in the entire world.

I felt that I had to settle in Seattle, a city I'd visited previously. Many people there were interested in whole-person healing. At first, I shared homes with new friends until I could get established. I struggled to become known, giving lectures and following up with people referred to me. It was a challenging time, but one beautiful morning when I turned on the radio, all my uncertainty melted away. I was listening to a talk on human energy fields presented by Valerie Hunt, a University of California researcher with advanced degrees in psychology and physiology. My heart raced.

In her laboratory at UCLA, Dr Hunt and her assistants used instruments developed by the National Aeronautics and Space Administration (NASA) to measure the body's electrical activity. She discovered that, "Although composed of the same electrons as inert substances, the human field absorbs and throws off energy dynamically. It interacts with and influences matter." Measuring various systems in the body, she found that each person has a unique energy field that shows where energy flows more freely while others are blocked. Significantly, she discovered that "changes occurred in the field before any of the other systems change."

"I can no longer consider the body as organic systems or tissues," she went on, "the healthy body is a flowing, interactive electrodynamic energy field."

I raced out after the program and purchased her very

helpful book, *Infinite Mind: Science of the Human Vibrations of Consciousness*, which featured an abundance of charts showing the shape of waves in the energy field that her laboratory instruments had recorded. I cannot begin to tell you how excited I was to recognise that Dr Hunt's work would make a huge difference in my healing techniques.

In the earliest days of my healings, when clients asked me whether I was working with their auras, I'd said yes. I was even standing them against a dark backdrop to see the light emanating from them. As it turned out, Hunt had studied various cultures that worked with the aura, chi, prana, life force, or odic force and observed that they were all referring to the human energy field — aura is an old term for this field. However, I'd always known intuitively that my work was beyond chakra work, which is generally considered as part of aura readings. The chakra concepts do not mesh with the healing lessons coming through to me. I do not use my hands and my work is more intensive than aura healers in significant ways. For example, I can actually readjust the frequency pattern of fields for maximum energy input into the body.

My time in Seattle was off to a very auspicious start. My confidence grew with my new knowledge that in at least one respected laboratory, scientists were doing work that corroborated my own intuitive findings about the human body and energy field. I must admit, it had been difficult to hold my beliefs close to my heart no matter how critics might insult me, but now I knew I was on solid ground. Dr Hunt's work didn't tell me anything I hadn't known already, but I felt much more comfortable having heard it from a scientist.

This was a turning point for me. Perhaps it was my new level of confidence that attracted clients to my door. Soon I could handle more complex cases and in fact, began reaching into higher spiritual dimensions to heal.

Chapter Two

Mother Nature's University

The Pacific Northwest captured my heart with its tall cedars, snow-capped mountains, bubbling streams, and abundance of wildlife. I lived in Seattle, a major city where residential streets are lined with trees and a park is always close by. I shared a house with charming roommates and felt at home in many ways. But not quite. Deep inside, I yearned for a serene and beautiful atmosphere that would nurture my blossoming healing abilities. An ideal home was waiting for me somewhere, I was sure, but I had no clue how I'd find it or afford it once found. Was it just wishful thinking on my part? I needn't have worried, as destiny was at work.

My client and friend Joel was aware of how difficult it was for me to share living space with other people. As much as I liked my roommates in Seattle, I was incredibly sensitive to any small patch of physical or psychic negativity and was always expending energy to keep my living space pristine. Clearing negative frequencies from everyone and everything could be a drain, and I needed to keep my energy pure for my work as a healer.

Joel had come to me a few months earlier in hopes of finding relief from pain in his back that he'd endured for years in spite of the best efforts of several health practitioners. He was absolutely thrilled with his newly painless spine.

In return, Joel did something special for me by suggesting that I look at a house belonging to his friends Jack and Merle. The house was empty, as his friends had recently moved out and had not decided whether to rent or sell. I was working on a donation basis and was concerned that it would be too expensive. Joel spoke with the owners and arranged for me to pay low rent and give healing sessions to Merle if I decided to move in.

I was so excited I barely slept the night before we were scheduled to see the place. Joel picked me up the next afternoon for the 90-minute drive south to the Olympia area. Beautiful Mt. Rainier, an almost perfectly conical volcano, formed an impressive backdrop for this pretty capitol city of Washington State on the shore of Puget Sound. At Olympia, we turned off the freeway and followed a tree-lined road along a bay covered with sailboats small and large. Here and there, verdant pastures were dotted with grazing cattle. Everything I saw filled my soul with joy.

"Here we are," Joel said as he turned left at a white mailbox and headed down the short dirt road that led to the house. I could almost hear the tall fir trees saying "Welcome to our forest Robyn, we will take care of you." Growing amid these magnificent trees were the tallest of foxgloves in vivid shades of purple, yellow, blue, white and mauve. Here and there were fallen logs covered in carpets of soft velvet moss. The site was enchanting.

The brown cedar house took my breath away. Perched on a bluff overlooking a teal blue bay, it was an architecturally interesting split-level with not one room square or rectangular. Tall windows in almost every room framed beautiful views of the bay. As an added bonus, most of the furniture was built in, so I wouldn't have to spend money I didn't have buying essential pieces. I loved the house so much, I would gladly have slept on the floor, but was happy I wouldn't need to do so. Without hesitation, I thanked Joel profusely and told him I would like to move in.

This would become my university; here the ailing bodies would communicate to show and teach me, not books or cadavers. Here I would also face my last remaining fear of living in a house by myself, especially one so far from town and neighbours. Yes, this house would work for me on many levels. With their pure vibrations, the woods and clean air would help strengthen my work and with my new strength I could easily clear any negativity that might be lingering there from Merle's illness. It was 1996 and I could see myself living here for years.

The next day I met the owners, a lovely couple, and signed the necessary agreement. I honestly believed that a miracle had made this house mine and I elevated Joel to "ground angel" status for finding the place for me and negotiating such a favourable price. I could never have done it without him. That night I luxuriated in my new home. It had been a long, long time since I had known that feeling.

On my first day in residence, I ran around buying staples and arranging my closets. Late in the day, I sat alone staring out at the sun setting over the waters of the Sound, reliving the incident that had nearly overwhelmed me just one short year earlier when I'd first returned to Seattle from Australia.

I had been deeply relaxed when my mind reached a state of profound silence and my soul had a chance to speak. In this deep state of knowing, I'd heard that I had a mission to introduce a new and different healing method to the world. I remembered shedding copious tears, feeling shock, disbelief, and most of all the seriousness of my responsibility. I'd also been informed of details about my brother's death and other events, all of which occurred during the following year, just as that voice inside had predicted. Now my sense of wonder was tempered by measurable progress I'd made with my healing abilities. Here I was, sitting in a beautiful little corner of heaven that had seemingly fallen into my lap. Clearly this was to be the place where healing lessons would deepen every day. I felt peaceful and fulfilled.

Next day, the mood shifted when a client named Milly came to see me. Unfortunately, she took it upon herself to interject a note of negativity the minute I opened the door "Robyn, you can't live all this way out on your own, you're so vulnerable as a woman alone."

"Please don't worry, I'll be okay! I'm protected," I said a little shakily.

She wouldn't let up. "Robyn, you need a gun. I'll lend you a double-barreled shotgun. It's easy to handle. You have to have protection."

I couldn't even think of having a gun in my possession. Even the thought terrified me as guns are banned in Australia. It's so different in the States where you can walk into any gun shop and purchase a lethal weapon. Milly was not about to take no for an answer and arrived the next day with the gun. It was so huge and heavy, I shook looking at it but she wouldn't leave until I let her show me how to shoot. I felt very uncomfortable having it in the house. I put it under the bed and found myself awake all night listening for noises and mentally going through lock and load lessons just in case. Wherever you live in the woods, there are plenty of mysterious night noises, so I got no sleep at all.

Next day, I phoned Milly to come collect the firearm, thanking her kindly and reassuring her I would be okay.

I must admit that the incident left me with some residual fear about things that go bump in the night. I was happy to have my breathing technique at the ready during the following months to reprogram those negative thoughts and feelings. As you can imagine, a lot of breathing went on in that house until I adjusted to being alone in the woods at night.

In *Conversations with the Body*, I gave directions for my Breath of Life technique. It's quite simple and effective, but you must be vigilant and use it right away when fear or other negative thought or emotion threatens to overwhelm you. You simply take a deep breath through the nose and hold it for a count of eight. While holding your breath, mentally recite an affirmation that directly contradicts your fear. In this case I repeated to myself, "I'm safe and secure." Then quickly blow out the breath through your mouth. Repeat the process eight or ten times. You can reprogram any negative thought or feeling with this technique if you catch it within twenty seconds.

Word of mouth spread very quickly about my form of healing, and clients came. Many thought nothing of making the long drive from Seattle to experience my healing sessions. The work was to evolve as their bodies presented more and more complex ailments. I was also finding new clarity when seeing inside these bodies.

It was anything but a clear day when Grace came to see me. The gloom of her mood matched the dark forbidding clouds threatening to burst with rain. Her body was so wracked with pain that I had to help her from her car into my living room where I had two chairs at the ready, facing out over the bay. At that time all of my healing sessions were performed in side-by-side chairs, with the client on my right.

Grace was a very troubled person, full of bitterness about a divorce. After more than thirty years of marriage, her husband had abandoned her for the proverbial younger woman. Grace had been a trusting wife and had no idea that his late nights at the office were actually spent with his new lover. She was shaky, very nervous about life in general and specifically about what I was intending to do.

I explained to her how I work, "First I scan your energy field."

"Do you mean my aura?" she asked. It's a common misnomer first-time clients use.

"It once was called the aura, Grace. But technically it's the electrical energy that extends out from our physical bodies. In all of my healing sessions, I first clear the energy field of negativity, which looks very much like TV snow. Apparently TV and radio interference is virtually identical to our field."

She nodded her understanding. I went on, "Then I look for body weaknesses, diagnosing them by finding weak circuits. As we progress with early sessions, I will repair these weak circuits, which, in turn, will bring your body to wellness."

Grace sighed, signaling that she was beginning to relax a bit, and I went on, "When your field is clear, I then envision the inside of your body, one quadrant at a time. First I scan your lower left side from the ground to your elbow," I said. "From there I go all the way up to the top of your head, then down the right side of your upper body ending with the lower quadrant, and back to the ground. Then I work using my energy ray by entering your crown."

Grace nodded again to indicate she was tracking with me.

"I tend to the weakened body parts that show in your field, strengthening your entire body. The engine that is the human body is incredibly complex and all of its parts need to be in harmonious working order. If any organ or system is out of synch, the entire body can stop working. Just think of the inner workings of your car; if one part fails, the car won't run."

My words had calmed Grace's nerves and she seemed ready to commence. I taught her the easy three-step Breath of Life process: inhale, count to eight, exhale strongly. I begin all of my sessions this way, helping my clients relax and centre. I took a Breath of Life too, though in recent years, I haven't needed to do so. My energy ray is ready at will.

"Now close your eyes, Grace. Tell your mind to stop for awhile, just put aside all thoughts."

As she drifted into deep relaxation, I was not surprised to see that her energy field was completely snowed. Yes, I literally see the field and the inside of the body with my eyes closed.

I cleared the negativity using my energy ray at full force, holding it with extreme concentrated focus against the negative power in order to destroy it. My positive energy has to be three times as powerful as the negative force in order to counteract and overcome it. I know when I've succeeded when I see dark snowy energy, the negative frequencies, lift off and float away, disempowered.

As I scanned through her body, I could see that Grace's pain stemmed from her liver. The emotion of bitterness caused liver malfunction and poisons had backed up in her body from acid thoughts directed against her husband. The tissues of the liver had actually tightened up, which affects its detoxifying function.

Grace's heart was also in trouble, its arterial tissues thickened. Acid from the liver was also affecting her bones. Ten years of obsessive negative thinking had brought about the arthritis that was causing her such pain.

I said, "Grace, I can help your body, but you are the only one who can control your negative thinking. You're destroying your body with it, but it's not hurting your ex at all. What you're doing just doesn't make sense." She looked at me quizzically, finding it hard to comprehend what I was saying.

"You must forgive and move on. When you have negative thoughts, replace them quickly by thinking positive thoughts about your two lovely children who love you very much. They could not have entered this lifetime through any other parents. Unfortunately when your job of procreation and parenthood was done, things changed. You now have to free yourself from the bondage of your own mind to stop producing poison and let your body heal."

Thank goodness Grace had taken no drugs for her condition, which made my job easier. Sometimes it takes awhile to wean the body from chemicals. I explained that her thoughts had blocked her heart generator from producing the love frequency needed to create a positive energy field, so necessary for a happy and healthy life. I knew she was motivated and hoped she would follow through by controlling her mind; I would do my part healing her body.

She did well, as it turned out. It took awhile to create a healthy shift in Grace's physical and emotional state. Eventually she became a new person, once again running on love power. In her note of thanks she wrote, "How could I have forgotten how to love for so long no matter what had occurred in my life? Thank you for introducing me to the purity of unconditional love."

My sessions tend to bring negative emotions to the surface to be dealt with and healed. By keeping clients linked to the beautiful higher dimensions where love and forgiveness abide, their negative emotions become easier to eradicate. In Grace's case, she had spent years in the dark valleys of the fourth spiritual dimension, which is hell in the literal sense. When she was released, true healing began in earnest and she moved toward the unconditional love of the fifth dimension. (I discuss dimensions in Chapter 12.)

Fighting through dark clouds of negative energy that shroud some clients takes considerable work on my part. I must keep my own vibrations pure and rhythmic and my field clear. I found it difficult to spend time in most places where people gathered. Going to movies was no longer much fun, for example, as I had to use a great deal of energy to keep my surroundings free of all negativity.

Here, overlooking Puget Sound, I found plenty of allies. Soon after I moved into my dream house, wild creatures gathered around. My energy has always attracted animals and birds wherever I've lived. Rac and Coon were male and female raccoons who came for their supper every evening and I fed them as if they were dogs, each in its own bowl. Raccoon Restaurant expanded when they arrived one evening with two babies. My menagerie included a beautiful fox I called Foxy who became very trusting. On his daily visits, he'd proudly stand near the bridge over a gully in front of my door, showing me his catch of the day. It was fascinating to observe his behaviour as he stood holding a poor small creature in his mouth for sometimes five minutes.

Many hummingbirds also visited. I'd never seen them before in my life, though they're common in the Pacific Northwest. Their energy output amazed me, their tiny wings beating so fast they were invisible. Other very vocal birds settled in the trees surrounding the house, serenading me morning and night. The wholesome environment of my new home was appealing and clients looked forward to driving down to see me.

Nora was a charming eighty-five-year-old woman, whose heart needed some very serious work. Her husband's death after fifty-five happy years of marriage had taken a huge toll. The tissues of her heart were weak as were the heartstrings, and her artery walls had thickened. Nora's angina pain was almost constant, a very dangerous state of affairs. She had avoided seeing physicians because of "...The way they treated George, they wouldn't allow him to die with any dignity."

Her age and the depth of her heartache concerned me. Basically, Nora was placing complete responsibility for her life on my shoulders. At the beginning of a session, I asked her to visualise the divine white light, which had previously been difficult for her. "We are going to try something new today to help you see the light, Nora," I said. "As you know, I don't want you to visualise darkness, even at night. Just close your eyes and imagine a huge light bulb shining brightly. Can you see that?"

"Oh yes," she said, "the white glow is lovely. I can

definitely see it." Nora didn't have to struggle to picture white light this time. Most clients had trouble visualising with closed eyes, so I was happy that my new idea had made a difference.

Nora interrupted my thoughts. "Now dear, would you like me to put a shade on that?"

There I was ready to go into session in all seriousness, and I wanted to break into giggles. I took it as a message to put a sense of humour into my work, which I do to this day. The bodies I'm working on love it and respond accordingly. Making healing fun lightens up the atmosphere and helps counteract the weightiness of illness. In ten sessions with Nora, I was able to stretch her arteries, reset the valves, and strengthen her aorta. The tissues and heartstrings strengthened wonderfully, leaving Nora looking fifteen years younger.

I also discovered that when my work became cheerier, I began to make friends with other people who were dedicated to living in a positive way, and my home became the venue for many playful get-togethers. My friends and clients were openminded evolved people, and their support helped enormously in the development of my abilities.

Toward the end of the first year in Olympia, I gave two lectures in Seattle that brought many new people to my door. One day, I took on thirteen suffering people — too many for my own good. That night, too exhausted to cook or even eat, I dozed off on the floor and slept there all night.

It was a good lesson for me to pay attention to my own needs. I was still tired when I made my annual Christmas trip to Australia. Exhausted, I could barely converse with my family.

On my return to Seattle, I decided to start charging a minimal fee, as donations were not even paying my living expenses. I had fought the idea of charging for healing for years until Jo and Derek, a married couple who were coming for healings, told me that they were paying more than fifty thousand dollars annually for supplements they'd been told to take by a natural health practitioner.

"Robyn, if you can heal us, look at how much money we'll save."

I couldn't believe my ears. Next day they carried in a box full of bottles of pills and capsules to show me. They were expected to take three handfuls daily. How could they even calculate the daily doses? I could not understand how anyone acting as a healer could expect a body weakened by ill health to process so many pills.

Before long, our sessions brought Derek and Jo to a high level of health and they were able to cut their huge doses to one multi-vitamin with minerals, with some extra Vitamin C, zinc, and Vitamin E along with fish oil for those important omega 3s. In my opinion, this is enough supplementation for most well bodies regularly supplied with organic food and pure water. I also recommend that those with troubled livers take milk thistle annually, a herb that specifically strengthens that overworked organ. Taking milk thistle one month per year is a good preventive dose — those with liver trouble can take more.

A member of International Assembly of Spiritual Healers & Earth Stewards, an exclusive worldwide association of healers and ministers, contacted me with an invitation to join their group. I was happy to learn that the group's stated intention was almost identical to my own: "...to render the utmost respect for the integrity of all individuals, whether or not human, and support the holistic integration of all human communities within the natural ecological ecosystems of the planet, solar system, galaxy and universe. ...To dispel, through both reasoned and intuitive knowledge, the ignorance that breeds fear, needless cravings, anger, rage, hatred, starvation, suffering, illness, abuse, cruelty, neglect, guilt, disease and wasting of life."

When I decided to join, several officers and members of the group travelled to my house to perform a moving ordination ceremony complete with candles and incense, certifying me as a Spiritual Healer and Earth Steward. This was important to me. I'd been christened in the Church of England at birth, which I felt totally comfortable with. I also wanted affiliation with and recognition by those who practised a broader based religion that was closer to my evolving spiritual sensibilities.

I felt that the religions most of us grew up with have not

kept pace with our expanding intelligence and intuition. Our knowledge of God and the universe has increased; animals and everything else on the planet have evolved. The world is changing, but so many people are clinging to the past that their vibrations are blocking the future of our planet. Fear of change is the key factor. But change will occur with them or without them. Hopefully, change will come in a gentle way, not through war and social upheaval. Democratic countries can show the rest of the world the way out of poverty and bondage — if only we will. It's good to keep an optimistic attitude and hold a positive intention for the evolution of our species and all others.

I grew in my knowledge of medical conditions and terminology, thanks in part to my acquaintance with a Seattle area physician named Dr John Walck MD. He was interested in several "alternative" modalities and was pleased with the results of healings I performed on some patients he'd referred to me. We've been friends for years now. He still sends some of his patients to me and is there for me when I need someone to clarify medical issues. Of course, I've referred clients to him and to other physicians around the world.

We all have those days when conventional medicine is exactly what we need. Doctors perform intricate surgeries that save people's lives, bind up wounds, set broken bones in a hurry, and perform many necessary and successful procedures. It's the unnatural chemicals in drugs that in my opinion do so much body damage. Many drugs only numb us, masking the real problem. In my experience, a numb body part lacks the power to heal. You might as well say to it, "You are so useless, you can't even do your job, take this pill."

In contrast, vibrational work empowers the body part. I say, "I'm here to help you. I know you are not doing well with that negative chemical invasion. We will work to remove it, then I will regenerate you to your glorious self." I reach out to their innate intelligence, communicating wellness by means of love.

As I see it, conventional medicine is from the outside in, my work is from the inside out. We are vibrational electrical beings, and the healing I do is very comfortable, non-invasive and compatible with the natural systems. In a sense, it brings the body back into harmony with itself.

As the learning went on at my private university, I gradually became aware that a major shift was taking place in my life, one that would set the tone for my work from then on, in a deep and profound way. I realised that I was now thinking from my heart. It was strange to find that my thoughts were not in my head, but came from what I can only describe as a well of warmth in my chest. I had learned years earlier at a Siddha Yoga Ashram in Australia to concentrate on the heart if you want to get things done in this world, and now my thoughts and feelings seemed to have merged, to have become one. This unity of heart and mind seems to be closer to Divine energy than anything I'd experienced before. It was the beginning of my rising through higher spiritual dimensions.

My heart had a kind of musicality about it. I would be deep in session and my heart would be singing a favourite song. It seemed to help the work. I've always believed that filling your atmosphere with beautiful music is an important way to keep your vibrations cycling at a high level. I suggest that you keep music on when you're away from home to help to clear the space. Nothing's as sweet as walking into high vibrational energy upon your return.

During those years in the woods, I tried to regenerate some ailing parts and tissues with a certain amount of success. This thrilled me. One client's finger had begun to re-grow, affirmed by his amazed physician. I wondered what the limits of regeneration might be. I was soon to learn in an unexpected way.

Julie came for sessions after I had successfully healed her daughter. Julie's thyroid gland had become cancerous and had been surgically removed. Her daughter wanted me to check her out to make sure she was still well, as it had been two years since the removal. During our second session I went deep into the area where the gland had been and noticed a very small section of healthy cells.

"Julie," I said, "I believe I may be able to re-grow your thyroid, as there is still some life there." A frightened look came over her face, "Just think about it," I added. "It's such an important gland to the body, it would be wonderful if you didn't have to take medication for the rest of your life."

The next day, Julie called to say she would not be continuing with her sessions. She did not want her thyroid back because of all the pain it had put her through. It was a good lesson for me to see the limits some clients place on themselves. I might have been able to stimulate the remaining thyroid cells to grow but could not force Julie to love her body enough to try. She blamed the gland, not her inability to get over an unsuccessful relationship, which had been the underlying cause of her disease. Holding negative thoughts and feelings had lowered her vibrational level and had affected her thyroid. The throat is our emotional area; the thyroid gland is connected to our ability to release emotions that no longer serve us.

Julie put a limit on her healing, but I was soon to encounter a woman who refused to believe in any kind of limitation. A friend called and asked me to heal someone by phone. Her friend was the mother of a famous vocalist, one of my favourite singers. She had heard about me and hoped I could assist her. The problem was, she had taken ill on a visit to Australia. I'd had success by phone before with the occasional client but they had been close by, not thousands of miles away. This would definitely be "remote healing," and I was not sure it would be successful. But I would give it a try. We had two sessions on the phone and achieved the desired result. I was surprised at how comfortable it felt and how well I could see inside her body. This opened up possibilities for me, but I did not know at the time that healing only by landline telephone would one day become the centre of my work.

Chapter Three
Bodies Reveal Their Secrets

My abilities have been evolving since the beginning of my healing journey in 1979, when I eradicated a tumour in my uterus before it could be surgically removed. My method is not static. Continuous improvement of my abilities has led to a verified success rate of more than ninety percent. I feel humbled by the responsibility, by the confidence my clients have in me, and by being chosen by a higher power to spread the word about these new dimensions in healing.

I learn from every client and sometimes seemingly inconsequential things produce big improvements in my work. Initially, I started sessions seated beside my clients, with them on my right. Then, while visiting another city, the layout of my hotel room necessitated seating the woman who'd come to see me on my left. The work remained essentially the same at the outset of the session when I closed my eyes and visualised her energy field. I went quadrant by quadrant, starting at the bottom left foot, up to the elbow region, then on up to the top of the head, coming down on the right side. I removed negative frequencies, repaired and strengthened circuits and diagnosed this woman the same as I always had done. When I repair and strengthen circuits I am actually replacing frequencies that have dropped out of their position in the circuit. Only when they remain in their correct position can that circuit work correctly.

When it was time to view the inside of her body, my vision was quite different from all previous sessions. Her body appeared on my mental screen as if she were standing directly in front of me with her back toward me. I was both surprised and pleased with this new development. My inner healer had known exactly what to do, presenting me with a vision of a body from a different angle than the one I was accustomed to seeing. This was not something I consciously thought about or decided to do. In fact, I was amazed to see a body from the back rather than from the side. It was a gift, as I'd never before had such a clear view of body parts. Since then, every person I work on shows up on my mental screen in the same way. Every advance that comes about in my work occurs as a sort of evolutionary change. I don't have to think about it, it just happens.

Seeing the Brain

When I enter a body, I begin at the fontanel at the top of the head where I check for any damage to the right and left hemispheres of the brain and alignment of head plates. These may be out of alignment if birth was difficult or if head injuries were sustained in an accident. Then I perform any neurological work necessary. At the front of the fontanel I can see a band of neurons that hold information relating to the person's birth.

The fontanel is left open at birth to receive Divine energy. Babies receive massive doses of unconditional love from above, which they need in order to develop their energy fields adequately. Love is every bit as important to babies as food is. Without it, many fail to thrive and some even die. Newborns radiate glowing pink energy. People goo and gaa around them because of the huge doses of love surrounding the baby.

When looking around inside bodies, I use my ray as an endoscope, but unlike the medical instrument, it is not solid, so I can get around corners. As you probably know, an endoscope is a small camera attached to tubing that physicians use to look inside the body.

Pituitary Gland

After checking for neurological problems, I then visit my favourite body part, the fingernail-sized pituitary gland situated near the base of the brain. It is commonly called the master gland, but I call it Captain Pituitary. It secretes hormones that help control major functions such as growth, blood pressure and metabolism and takes on major responsibility for the body's wellness and emotional happiness. This gland contains the early psychological and health history of the person up to the age of seven. I can tell clients quite a lot about themselves by reading it.

In many people, the pituitary reveals fear of the dark in infancy, an understandable condition considering that we lived in a world of bright light prior to entering the womb. A child might also have been afraid of noise and of adults, who looked like giants through baby's blurred vision. Sometimes, especially in the beginning of work with a new client, the pituitary is very shy, which indicates the personality of the person as a small child. Conventional wisdom tells us that you have only the first seven years of a child's life to help them develop their personality. I don't doubt the truth of that.

The pituitary communicates in a childlike manner, often using baby talk. It might tell me, "I'm tired." I have come to recognise this as a statement that the entire body is tired, not just the gland. If it says, "I'm sick", it's also speaking for the total body. The pituitary can communicate in pictures as well as speech. I see little girls who want to be fairies holding out their dress and dancing with a wand. Little boys might be climbing trees and playing with their pet animals. This gland seems to only carry the positive memories of childhood. Rarely have I seen damage to a pituitary, though it's often underdeveloped. On two occasions this brave little gland told me of its owner's death wish.

As clients become well, their self-assurance increases,

often to higher levels than ever before. Their new confidence is directly related to the strengthening I've given the pituitary. If a client returns for a tune-up session after months or even years, I get an exuberant welcome from this gland. I am always delighted with the cheery greeting this body part gives me as it recognises that I'm helping it do its job. My friendship with these precious little glands has provided me with ever-deeper understanding of their complex workings.

I believe that all body parts have responsibility for playing their role for body function because they are pure positive energy. They are fed only the Divine love energy. The only negative that can be attached to them is the invasion of any illness, an illness that has derived from negativity in the energy field.

Immune System

After I check the pituitary, the next port of call is the immune molecule, located very deep in the left hemisphere of the brain approximately centre-crown. This is a large L-shaped molecule that gives information to me about the immune system. If it is straight up and down like the back of this L, all is well; if it slants down at an angle, I know that cancer has entered the body. More often than not, it is drowned in inflammation because of mobile phone use. During sessions, I clean the area around it and then lengthen the long side of the L. Then I can see whether it has shrunk, which indicates the person is very ill or is using antibiotics.

Of all of the visions of the body that I shared in *Conversations with the Body*, this molecule is the hardest for people to understand. How could I see a molecule? I was pleased to read about the 2006 Nobel Prize winner in chemistry, Roger Kornberg of Stanford University, who received the prize for his work in identifying the huge RNA polymerase molecule that consists of many thousands of atoms. Kornberg, like other scientists, visualised what his theoretical assumption might look like before he actually identified it. According to an October 2006 article from Reuters, "Kornberg made an image of a molecule that RNA uses to read and transcribe the DNA code into something that actually works. Kornberg's team set out to visualise this structure. When Roger Kornberg started working on it, it was so complicated, some people thought he was somewhere between ambitious and crazy to try to solve its structure…" Though this molecule may not be the same one I see, there's a chance that it is. What's indisputable is that the process of visualisation scientists use is remarkably similar to mine.

The majority of people use one side of their brain more than the other. Inflammation is a huge problem in brain function and it's been getting worse in recent years as mobile phone use increases. Nine out of ten brains I look at today are flooded with inflammation. Negative frequencies from mobile phones fuse with frequencies in human energy fields, causing blockage in the field, then blockage in the head's fluid flow. Circulation of head fluids slows down and can stop for a short time. Once I drain the fluid, brains become clean enough for me to reset the electrical flow between the neurons. To use a visual description, if you placed your hands, thumb to thumb, in the centre of the hypothalamus at the back of the neck, then fanned the fingers to meet on top of the crown, this is the passageway of the electrical flow. I am now able to bypass the electrical hemisphere pathway if there is an area in the brain too damaged to reinstate.

As my work evolves, I can detect more detail in the human brain and can identify foreign growths with more clarity. These range from soft tissue tumours to hard gristle-like tumours to growths very similar to warts. I remove all growths and their root systems, which is delicate work as their roots can be amazingly long.

I have identified old skull fractures that doctors had failed to notice after accidents and have been able to move head plates for alignment if need be. This is not accomplished overnight. It's difficult work that requires quite a number of sessions.

My work in the brain usually brings about more balanced hemispheres, which are now working electrically, leading to clarity of thought and sharpness of memory. The effect on a person's function after I accomplish this is amazing. Eyes that have not been working together as a team now become stronger. Of course, I have prepared them by cleaning and strengthening them during each and every session.

In my view, our brain is an electrical processor and transformer. It processes all learned information but does not contain it. The information is transformed into the computerisation system in our energy field. I have no doubt that it controls our motor skills and senses. The computer holds knowledge while the brain operates our senses and motor skills and is attuned to our emotions. The brain does not respond to pain; the Egyptians were the first people known to perform surgery without numbing the site.

Eyes

I then continue my healing pathway down the front of the head to the eyes. First I clear out inflammation and drain infected fluids from behind them. This process can continue for some time when working in a head with neurological problems. Eyes are not able to function effectively if the head is not free of impurities. I check for cataracts and any "spots before the eyes" that are virtually impossible to remove any other way. I then work on the optic nerves at the back and sides, cleaning then strengthening them with my energy tool.

Over time, I perceived that the eye doing most work would start to rest as the weaker eye strengthened. This is amazing because the strong eye knows when it's time for this action and can judge when it is needed. As I see it, they communicate this need to each other. All body parts that come in pairs exhibit this tendency to work together in some coordinated way, depending upon the needs of the particular body. It's been an exciting discovery. I might suggest eye exercises to my clients to help the eyeballs work in concert.

I became increasingly deft at changing the shapes of my energy tool; I can use it in a sweeping action like a broom, as a hook to pull out infection, and as various sizes of spheres, the finest to clear the eye tear duct. I can also use it as a very fine scalpel for dissections. Cataract removal usually takes two to three sessions.

Sinuses

Our very important sinus systems are having difficulty now because of pollution and shallow breathing. The colour of infections that I clear away from sinus cavities indicates the length of time they've been there — some for many years. I find that frequent use of my three-step Breath of Life technique by the client helps me to clear sinuses. Drainage can take quite some time. As sinus cavities drain, my clients often think they have flu symptoms.

When you think about it, life has become so easy, we only push buttons and don't take deep breaths unless we make a special effort. I can remember as a child watching granny

Penny do the family washing, scrubbing furiously on a glass washboard, puffing and panting, perspiring profusely in the steamy laundry. Using modern conveniences all day leaves our respiratory systems underutilised and weakened.

Throat

After I clear sinuses, I move to the throat. Here I pay special attention to the thyroid gland, which has to be strong and well balanced to harmonise with the upper lymphatic team and the heart. If it's very ill, I prepare it for regeneration, which is a huge part of my work. Thyroid glands are very amenable to my work. They communicate with me by silently conveying their emotions rather than words. Most thyroid glands are in trouble now. These beautiful glands are very attached to our emotional being, which is the throat area. Once people release troublesome emotions to free themselves from bondage, thyroid glands take on a very healthy look and may even increase in size. I'm fascinated that this gland is shaped like a butterfly, ready to fly when its owner is able to let go of old hurts.

Lymphatic System

The lymphatic team on both the right and left side of the upper body region is next. Often lymph nodes or other parts of the lymphatic system are blocked. This immediately tells me that their owner has been having trouble accepting an occurrence in his or her life. Something is keeping them from going with the flow and they're putting on the brakes, causing the drains to block. These sensitive little glands love to be loved and talked to in baby talk. I'll say, "Come on little darlings, it's okay, you're all right!" It's amazing how quickly they will release and flow again. It's important to keep your lymph system flowing and in complete harmony with the thyroid gland and heart, especially if you are suffering from elevated blood pressure.

Mouth

I check gums for bacteria, and then clean them out if needed. It is very common to find infections around tooth roots. My work is very effective for strengthening gum tissue and cleaning out bacteria and infection. I don't do a lot of work in the dental department, leaving that to holistic dentists.

Lungs

I enter the right bronchial tube next, looking for patches of poisoned or thickened tissue. If inhalation of noxious chemicals has poisoned the client, I pare the distressed tissue away. These patches continue to surface for many sessions, so it takes a bit of time to successfully eradicate all of the effects of poisoning. I use the same method of paring for tissue thickened by cigarettes or marijuana. If I see small valves at the top of bronchioles, it tells me that the client suffered from shortness of breath, especially as a child, which carried on into adulthood. My work and the client's constant breathing of the Breath of Life can expand them. The tissues here tell me if the person has smoked cigarettes or drugs, the lungs will also reveal this.

Virus infection of the lungs is widespread now. Viruses actually bury themselves in the soft tissue at the base of the lung and live a long time, eventually causing massive damage. A dry cough is usually the sign of their existence. In some cases I am able to drain off fluid through the bottom of the lung. I use this method with cancer clients' fluid. For most people, however, my work gradually brings infection in the lungs to the surface. After the first or second session, coughing up of congested material begins and continues until the lungs have cleared. Many clients report major coughing first thing in the morning and last thing at night to expel congestion.

I must explain that my work heals by surfacing any weakness in a body, lung congestion being the perfect example. Some people get boils and pimples for a short time as infections and impurities work their way out of the body. In some cases, a certain amount of discomfort occurs during the surfacing, but before long, the negative leaves and the positive takes over to create a kind of perfect health available only to bodies totally free from impurities.

Breasts

I move from the lungs to the chest wall, checking

breasts for any lumps. If I see even the slightest indication of cancer, I ask the client to see his or her doctor for testing. No matter where in the body I come upon a suspicious invasion of cancer-like cells, I apply the same principle. If medical testing reveals malignancy, my client then decides whether to proceed with conventional or natural healing.

Louisa, a client I helped through a near-death emergency after she was kicked in the liver by a horse (see Chapter 13) called a year after that incident saying she felt tired. My scan revealed a lump in her left breast, which neither she nor her husband was aware of. Though I thought it was benign, I suggested a medical scan to relieve any nagging doubt she might have about cancer as much as to confirm my findings. Louisa and her husband had complete confidence in my work from previous treatments, but followed my direction to get a scan. Tests revealed that my diagnosis was correct and also showed where I had been chipping away at the tumour.

During a follow-up phone call they told me that they'd related the incident to friends who refused to believe that I'd diagnosed a lump through the telephone lines even though it had been confirmed by medical testing. I suppose I should get used to it, but such negativity about my work always hurts. This work is as natural to me as breathing.

Heart

The beautiful heart is next. I start my work above the

heart in order to get a clear view of the cardiovascular system. If main arteries have tissues thickened by smoking or wear and tear, I don't pare them as I do with bronchial tubes, I stretch them. As I perform this action, I need to reset the valves to fit and also to retime them so that coronary circulation can take place unhampered. Re-strengthening the heart muscle is also necessary.

Hearts are happy about my work and usually cooperate fully. I love working with them. Readjusting valves is delicate and very artistic. I use my finest ray to do this work, using it to work around valves and stretch them until I have perfect flow. This might not happen immediately.

It's not uncommon to find small leaks in the upper valves, which I can close easily. It sometimes takes three or four sessions to succeed in this closure. I meet with resistance, however, if the client I'm working with has an emotional problem stemming from the heart, such as chronic worry about a loved one, and loss or lack of love. When the heart is overly protective of itself, it blocks my ray. I can only repair the heart if this client does not realise I'm working on the heart's rhythm. Amazingly, a heart has never spoken to me verbally. Hearts speak through the emotions.

Liver

Moving to the right I now get to the liver, which helps metabolise our food. It disperses a quart of bile daily, cleans the blood and is also a chemical factory. It stores chemicals needed from foods we have eaten. It's a marvelous regenerator even if 60 percent of its cells have been destroyed. Significantly, in this day of wanton drug overdoses, prescription as well as illegal, the liver breaks down toxic substances and medicinal products in a process called drug detoxification.

Most people's livers are working overtime, dealing with pollution, drugs, and other forms of poison. To make matters worse, in recent years, they have become riddled with viruses, worms and other parasites. Parasite power is on the rise as we import more farmed seafood from Third World countries and travel to far-flung outposts of civilisation. I discuss parasites in detail in Chapter 9.

If I see viruses or any type of parasite in the liver, I am allowed to kill them, which I do gladly. I use the ray to enter their labyrinths or homes, destroying viruses and hooking them out. To get rid of worms, I sweep back and forth with my ray to disturb and destroy them in both lobes of the liver if need be. I continue working over several sessions until I see no signs of life from the invaders. Sometimes in the first session there appear to be only a few. With the disturbance of my ray, I've been shocked to see so many in the second session. It's as though I've opened a can of worms — literally.

Huge amounts of infection pour out once the liver is cleaned up and strengthened. If the client is harbouring worms, I suggest a chemical dose to get rid of any leftover parasites. A back-up dose of medication is needed for complete eradication of eggs. Cleansing the ensuing infection from these invasions is a huge job, as it involves thoroughgoing trips through thirty-two feet of intestines over every session. Livers invaded by worms take a long time to heal as they are still trying to perform the huge amount of work they're responsible for.

Virus invasions are easier, but it still takes as many as four sessions to destroy them. Several clients suffered from more than one type of parasitic infestation that continued to cause havoc until all were eradicated. Once the liver is cleansed of worms, viruses and the infections they cause, I can regenerate it back to wellness.

If parasitic or viral invaders have been present in the liver for a significant period of time, the heart is weakened as well. When the heart receives impure blood from the infested liver, a sort of double whammy of distress occurs from both the infestation and from elevated levels of natural body tension because the sensitive heart knows it's in trouble.

Livers can also exhibit hardened tissue brought about by holding onto bitter emotions, usually about a difficult relationship. This will impair its output of bile, necessary for dissolving fats. Acidity then backs up in the body, often leading to arthritis and heartburn.

The liver is quite a character. I have seen it sulking if its owner has eaten something it doesn't like — frequently cheese or yogurt with preservatives. I love this wonderful organ that is the hardest worker in the human body. It's the start of the body's garbage disposal unit and inevitably the entire digestive system suffers if it is in trouble.

Livers seem to know that a session with me is on the schedule and many of them honour me by starting a strong detox process in the preceding 24 hours. It's as though they want to please me by appearing as clean as possible.

Gallbladder

The gallbladder is the teammate of the liver. This precious little organ is emotionally attached to a parent, usually the mother. If a client has been thinking negative thoughts about a parent, it will become upset. The gallbladder will never be happy unless parent issues have been resolved. Though my clients are usually in a deep state of relaxation during the healing sessions, I verbally encourage them to resolve their parent issues.

Gallstones are easy to remove. If very large, I can break them down to make their exit painless. Gallstones are prolific in any geographical area that has a large amount of lime scale in the water system. Lime can collect in the human body just as it does in washing machines, toilets and dishwashers. If you live where the water is overloaded with lime, such that you see the calcium-lime collecting on your faucets, please drink bottled water. Alternatively, you could filter the lime away with a good filter.

Sometimes the ducts between the liver and gallbladder malfunction. I have actually seen and straightened kinks in the ducts, and the valve systems often need adjusting.

Stomach

As the first part of the gastrointestinal tract, the stomach's job is to churn up the food into liquid, preparing it for treatment by the small intestine.

Vegetarians' stomachs are often in a terrible state, lacking tone and muscle due to lack of activity. Drinkers of strong tea and coffee have brownish stomach linings, dyed by these beverages. Ulceration may be present, which is fairly easy to fix. I keep cleaning the infection until nice healthy pink tissue emerges, which signifies that healing has occurred. Emotional anguish and incorrect diet are the main causes. Recently, I discovered that it is possible to reline stomachs.

I always make sure that the entrance to the intestine from the stomach is wide enough. If not, I enlarge it. Infections seem to gather here and this area attracts worms, another reason you need to ensure sufficient acid production. Enough acid will not allow anything foreign to grow. I regularly see roundworms and threadworms and their eggs here. Tapeworms show up too. They flatten themselves onto the wall with barbs. The only reason I pick them up is that my ray makes them move, otherwise their camouflage is so good they'd be impossible to find. I believe that's why medical scanning does not locate them.

Pancreas and Spleen

The pancreas, which secretes digestive enzymes and the hormone insulin, cannot function robustly if the liver and stomach are not strong. Once they become well it regenerates. The pancreas has been gradually strengthening as I work on the liver, gallbladder, stomach and spleen. Once the digestive system improves from the work, it quickly strengthens. It does not receive my ray generation and I know and respect this.

A troubled spleen can appear swollen and has a grey look, especially at the bottom. If really ill, the entire organ looks grey. The spleen takes on the emotional tone of the entire person. It won't accept my regeneration if its owner has an independent nature. Instead, it usually rejects my offer virtually stating, "No, I can do it myself!" It usually does too, once it gets the idea. It's fantastic to see the colour changes that occur as these body parts come into wellness.

Kidney and Bladder

I now move to the bladder and kidneys. Here I may encounter kidney stones, bacterial infection, and poorly functioning ducts and valves. I can see whether the person is drinking enough pure water by the relative cleanliness of these filters. Commonly, one kidney is larger than the other, which rarely means anything dangerous. I often run into a small group of cells, similar to a bunch of grapes, attached to a kidney. I see it as early kidney stone development. I dissect it to allow removal. No client has ever suffered pain as the stones were leaving, as I am able to smash the larger ones that might cause discomfort.

I used to "hitch up" bladders but as my work evolved I no longer had to do so, instead relining the bladder and strengthening muscle tone.

Reproductive System

In women, I make sure alignment of ovaries, womb and uterus is done, as this aids in comfortable menstruation. If a woman in her forties still wants to bear a child, I strengthen her remaining eggs. (In Chapter 7 I go into this process in detail.)

I'm always looking for growths, warts and infection. If I'm suspicious that cancer cells may be lurking I tell the client to have a medical checkup. Growths on ovaries are sometimes caused by the negative emotions of a woman who wants to prevent pregnancy. If she does not want a child, she uses this as a protective measure.

Prostate malfunction is the main problem I encounter in the male reproductive area and weakness in the bladder valves is very common. This means that they would have been bed wetters or hard to potty train. These valves can strengthen with maturity. However, the person will never know what it's like to have a strong direct flow of urine. They will have a lifetime of inconsistent flow. I believe this leads to prolific urination later in life and can be connected to prostate problems.

The walnut size shell surrounding the prostate gland can become contaminated and coagulated. I am able to clean the gland and its shell with success. The problem comes about mainly because the male has not ejaculated for many years, as he should. Most men are embarrassed when I tell them about it. In this case, phone work is better; the line between the client and myself is more open, so to speak. Infection can also gather behind the shell, where the duct exits. This requires constant cleaning over a series of sessions until eradicated. It's also interesting that males don't get embarrassed on the phone when I reach the penis area as they often do in person. They seem to think I'm not looking at size on the phone.

Colon

I often see infection in the ascending colon due to leaking and weakened tissue. Inability to express emotions or problems may bring about blockages of the colon, and males are the greatest sufferers. Those who have had colon surgery may have parts situated in the wrong places because surgeons stuffed healthy tissue back into the body cavity after examining them without regard for their previous placement. The confused body parts may function poorly, not knowing where they live anymore. I must stress the fact that every part of the human anatomy has its own space inside. Fortunately, I can realign parts, strengthen their tissue, and bring them back to full functioning, with, of course, the help of a good diet on the part of the client. Most clients are delighted to be able to put their laxatives aside now that they are making perfect stools after sometimes a lifetime of bowel trouble.

Another thing that I see in great numbers of people is a problem in the area where the ascending colon curves to become the transverse colon. Here the curve may be too acute, causing digestive slowdown. I am able to ease this curve so intestinal contents can flow smoothly. I actually go through the inside of the bowel all the way, removing polyps especially those that may be in the ascending colon. Hemorrhoids are easy to remove. Sometimes I find a tumour-like blockage during my internal scan, about five inches from the start of the ascending colon, which I remove.

Extremities

Knees are subject to injury from falls, sports, normal wear and tear, and from using the limb in unnatural movement to protect higher body parts that may be painful, especially in overweight people. I see pieces of bone and gristle floating around in many clients' knees. I don't always work on them, depending on their interference with activity.

Ankles and knees regenerate wonderfully well. It's amazing how many ingrown toenails I find. They respond when the owner cuts a V shape in the centre.

While working on legs, varicose veins improve. I clean hips of calcification and prepare them for regeneration. Often the ball joint is dry. I pull fluid down to oil them, so to speak.

After I finish with the legs, I then move back up to shoulders and arms to remove any acidity I see. Neck vertebrae slowly leak acid-like fluid if they've been out of alignment for a great length of time. It may then seep through the shoulders, causing havoc and pain in elbows and fingers. I clean up these areas with my energy ray relatively easily. I also clean the nerves at the top of the shoulders. Epsom salt baths help detoxify stuck acids in hands and feet, which occurs with gravitational drainage.

Spine

I work on spines during every session in an ongoing effort to keep them flexible and as strong as they can be. It's then time to work on the back, which is facing me in my visualisation. I check the hypothalamus area and then drain any build up of inflammation. It may be a residue from the previous session that's causing discomfort. I come down the neck vertebrae to straighten them, removing calcification, checking spaces between discs and vertebrae.

Ears

I go through the ear canal next, amazed at how many pierced eardrums I find. The scar tissue I encounter can usually be removed. If I find huge chunks of wax, I push them through. Old infection can be lurking here as well.

Women usually have keener hearing. This is the natural state, as we are on a higher vibration with ears made to hear our babies' cries. When our job of mothering is over, our vibration may lower.

More men seem to suffer deafness with maturity, possibly believing that they've heard everything they needed to know. Some mature women who have received my CD report not hearing it properly the first few times they play it. As it raises their vibrations, they hear it clearly. There may be an emotional connection as well, with the subconscious saying, "I won't listen; I don't want to hear it."

I continue down the spine doing the same as I did with the neck, paying special attention to the sciatic area. Tailbone realignment is common, as a great many people have damage in this area. I return to the top of the spine to go all through the bone marrow. If the consistency is uneven and contains areas of grey threads, the marrow is unwell. I create a mix, dragging healthy marrow into the ailing marrow. This can take several sessions but the results add greatly to health and well being.

Finally, I check the spinal cord and also review the

spinal nerves to make sure they are strong. If inflammation is present, I remove it so that each and every one of these sensitive threads has its own space, as it should. MS sufferers have thickened inflammation that ties up surrounding nerves at the top of the nerve column. I find it fascinating that most people diagnosed with MS are incorrectly labeled.

In the final sessions I can realign the skeletal structure. I do this by looking at the bones, repositioning any vertebrae that are out of alignment, almost as if I were placing my hands on either side of the spinal column and sculpting it into shape. I achieve this by visualising the client's skeletal structure, viewing it from the back. A great many spines tip to the right or left; very few are straight. I follow up by giving the spine a "power zap" with my energy ray to give it the energy it needs to stay in place. I achieve this by visualising the client's skeletal structure, viewing it from the back. This realignment process can take several sessions, with the reward a spine that again moves with fluidity and flexibility. Sometimes exercises are required to help the spine maintain its improved condition. If needed, I explain them to the client during the session.

Fountain of Youth

After each session, clients look as though they've had facelifts. The tissues have plumped and their faces glow. Skin is the last thing to permanently change in the healing process. Any body part that accepts regeneration becomes very youthful. I think of the vibration that I work with as the real fountain of youth.

My work is a two-way street, however. I make it very clear at the start that clients need to follow my advice to a tee so we don't have any setbacks. This does not always happen. You would be surprised how many forget to take the ten to fifteen breaths daily I encourage for oxygen, chest expansion, sinus clearing and glowing good health. "Have you done your breaths?" I ask at the beginning of each session. If the person forgot to breathe, I know this healing is going to be more difficult than it needs to be. Once a client takes responsibility, things go very well indeed.

Chapter Four
Fly to Emotional Freedom

My enchanting cedar house on the banks of Puget Sound continued to serve as my home and healing university for three wonderful years. Looking out at gentle ripples on the bay in front of my house, I felt in harmony with myself and all of nature. Tall cedars cast shadows on the water, catching the muted autumn light as the days became shorter. I could feel the enormity of Mt. Rainier as a magnetic force that grounded me. I experienced a new centredness in this northern place so far from the sun swept beaches and golden light of my Australian homeland. And at night, the shimmering moon seemed close enough to touch. Once again, I was living in a home where I could see the full moon from the living room, as though it were following me from country to country, always welcoming me home.

Clients presented me with hundreds of different conditions to heal and with only a few exceptions, my abilities somehow kept pace with their needs. Rarely was I presented with health problems I could not resolve and when I was, most of those clients were bogged down with emotional problems they were not willing or able to overcome. Over time, I became aware that almost all of the physical ailments people wanted me to heal were triggered by emotional problems.

I was surprised when a client named Lisa began to call me complaining of heart palpitations long after a successful healing. I thought she'd been maintaining her health, with old emotional problems taken care of. She had moved on from an unsuccessful relationship and I thought she was happy with a new man.

"Let's talk, Lisa. I'm picking up a mother problem. Am I correct?"

Lisa admitted that she and her mother were no longer speaking. "The first Christmas after my separation from Mike, she invited him for the day. No matter how hard I tried, she would not change her mind. She told me that her relationship with him was good I was the one having problems with him." By now Lisa was in tears. "I stayed home on Christmas," she sobbed, "as I felt mum was caring for my ex's needs, not mine."

I needed to give her some perspective in a hurry. "You're a mature woman, Lisa, and you need to make amends with your mother. It's breaking your heart and I cannot just go on re-attuning it. Don't you realise you are spiritually connected to her? You are a huge part of her life. She carried you and went through tremendous pain to get you here. You chose her as a parent for some reason and she is one of your strongest teachers."

By now Lisa had settled down. "Yes, I see your point Robyn. Thanks for reminding me. I'll give it a try." After another few sessions, Lisa reconciled with her mother and her heart was happy once again.

I saw a considerable difference in the emotional makeup of men and women. Virtually all of the men who came for healing participated in a straightforward manner and their bodies responded almost effortlessly. If I asked a man to breathe the Breath of Life twenty times a day, he did. Their energy fields might have shown murky areas of emotional upset prior to healing, but they cleared up satisfactorily with few recurring problems. They let go of old emotions easily.

Most of my clients were women, who were more likely to have serious emotional problems that persisted through several sessions and threatened their physical health. One woman was so crippled with anxiety that I had to go out in my driveway and do our session in her car — though nothing physical was curtailing her ability to walk.

During get-acquainted times with new clients, I always asked, "What emotional problem lowered the vibrations of your field allowing this physical condition to take hold? What brought it on?" In an amazing number of cases, women went back to their childhoods for their answers. As many as sixty-five percent cited physical and emotional abuse and even sexual molestation by a member of the family. They also mentioned troubled relationships with their husbands, children, or others they loved. For both men and women, some form of love gone wrong was the central issue.

Some men had suffered through abuse and rocky relationships, but they could more easily put the unpleasantness behind them and move on. A common emotional problem affecting huge numbers of men comes from their fathers expecting too much of them.

I found that most men believe their role in life is fairly simple. They may spend long hours working, but their energy is organised to go in a single direction. They just get on with the job. Perhaps they are good at denial as well. Women feel they need to be proficient at many things at the same time. They are expected to bear the children, hold down a job, keep the household running, and look their best all the while. Perhaps the twenty-first century will see a more equitable division of work.

Today, many young women in their prime childbearing years are opting out of motherhood, preferring a career. My generation was just expected to have children. Personally, I would not have missed having my adorable children for anything. Those were very happy years for me. I actually experienced motherhood from a very early age, caring for my brother and sister after my mother's death. It's not an easy job. I would certainly advise anyone who decides to bear children to take it very seriously. It's the most responsible thing you will ever take on. Evolution demands that our offspring attain one level of consciousness higher than ours.

In truth, no one has a perfect childhood or stress-free existence. We all have emotional scars and may become angry and depressed about not having enough love. Lack of love, repressed love, misplaced, distorted, misunderstood, unexpressed, unrequited love — the downside of love has endless varieties. Ninety percent of our emotional problems are about love. We yearn for perfect love and few of us know what it is, how to find it, or more importantly, how to give it. We need it, we want it, and without it we die. We've done some foolish things to "make" someone love us and we've unreasonably clung to a loved one long after the love has gone.

But things are looking up. Now, on my twelfth year of this journey, I am beginning to notice women making progress in the emotional area. They're taking charge and not allowing emotions to sink them. For one thing, they are getting smart about relationships. They're less likely to let men dominate them and are refusing to blame themselves for everything if things go wrong. Hopefully they are also expressing love in appropriate ways so that family members feel secure.

Emotional blockages are mainly caused by fear of flying, and I don't mean flying in an airplane. I mean taking charge of your life and becoming your best self. Fear is the opposite of love. When you learn to love yourself, you will be able to conquer fear.

If circumstances in your life make you unhappy, please go right ahead and make changes. If you don't like your home, move to one you do like. If your job is oppressive, find a new one. If your partner becomes nasty and threatens to leave, don't be afraid to say good-bye. If you have a general sense of unease, listen carefully to what your mind tells you first thing in the morning, even before you open your eyes. As a poet wrote, "the morning breeze has many secrets to tell you."

If you ask yourself just before you go to sleep at night, "What's bothering me? What emotional problem is lowering the vibrations of my field?" the still small voice of dawn will bring you the answer. Perhaps not on the first morning, but be persistent and the answer will surely come.

When you become aware of things that are troubling you, act quickly to free yourself from emotional bondage. Draw a clear line between this moment and every negative feeling and thought from the past that holds you in its grasp, depleting your energy. No matter what it is — regret, remorse, guilt, fear, sorrow, anger, despair, or anything else — own it and then release it immediately. If you continue to cling to the past, even unconsciously, no amount of my work or any other will give you total wellness. Until you find a way to rid yourself of unhappiness, this emotional problem will weaken the vibrational power of the circuits in your field and your body will suffer. I believe that women have a harder time than men do in this respect. We have been disempowered, for example, by being told by religions that we were made from a man's rib. We succumb to negative emotions because we don't believe we have the strength to overcome them. Women, particularly, become overwhelmed by their own limited ideas of who they are. Few people have told them how strong they are, instead there has been an almost concerted effort to try and keep women feeling needy in order to manipulate them. For example, frequent TV commercials for prescription drugs to solve all our problems underscore our weakness. It's our perceived weaknesses they play to, never our strengths.

Perhaps some people need drugs or therapy, but I do believe that great numbers of people can learn to work with their minds and emotions to direct them away from the negative and toward positive thoughts and feelings.

Start by replacing your negative "I can't" thoughts with a good strong "I can." "I can" is the very definition of self-esteem, sorely lacking in too many women. Improvements will come gradually for most people, but they will come if you keep at it.

This list will give you an idea of negative emotions and the positive emotions you can change them to:

FLY TO EMOTIONAL FREEDOM

NEGATIVE EMOTIONS	POSITIVE EMOTIONS
VICTIM, WOUNDED INNER CHILD, ADDICTIVE NATURE	HIGHER SELF, GOD ENERGY ACTING PURELY
Full of petty willfulness	Attuned to a higher will
Knows only a possessive allowing controlling kind of love	Loves unconditionally, allows others to have perfect freedom
Lies endlessly	Totally committed to the Truth
Takes himself/herself very seriously, cannot bear taunting or levity	Often uses humour to heal
Full of doubt	Full of faith
Thinks God can be manipulated with "good deeds" or the right prayers or lots of affirmations	Knows prayers, affirmations and deeds are to awaken awareness of the Divine within one's self
Believes the body is who we are	Knows we are Spirit only temporarily housed in a body
Self-destructive, compulsively drawn into behaviours that produce sickness and disease	Behaves with self-respect that produces wholeness of body, mind, and spirit
Feels undeserving of joy	Knows joy means a healthy connection to God and is everyone's right
Full of self-condemnation	Full of self-forgiveness and compassion
Concentrates on faults of others	Looks at own defects of character with compassion and forgiveness in order to heal them
Strives for instant fulfillment from things in the outer world	Knows that lasting fulfillment comes from the inner relationship with God
Hangs onto and nurtures resentment, bitterness and past wounds	Forgives others as readily as the self is forgiven, letting go of the past

Makes excuses and blames others for failure and all that's wrong in life	Looks at own contributions to events, brings own faults to the fore for forgiveness
Condemns self for having ordinary human weaknesses and desires	Knows that strength is gained by rising above weaknesses and desires
Facing failure, allows self to wallow in discouragement and despair	Knows that even in failure we are still infinitely loved, to rise and try again
Wears a mask, acts a part, tries to be all things to all people	Desires to be the true self, true to ourselves and speaking truth to others
Plans for fulfillment in the future	Knows that fulfillment is only in each moment, the present eternal Now
Procrastinates self-improvement	Starts self-improvement NOW, with baby steps if need be
Worries endlessly about the future, about all the "what ifs"	Knows that God and faith live in the eternal NOW
Boasts about self constantly	Knows that self-worth is internal and real, doesn't need to be proclaimed
Ruled by emotions, feels helpless over own feelings and emotions, can only react	Ruled by a sense of inner peace, able to act instead of just reacting
Uses emotions, (sulleness, anger moodiness) to control others	Prefers harmony and belongingness to a sense of control
Diverts attention from own inner pain and emptiness by creating chaos among others	So full of inner life that his/her very presence creates a feeling of harmony among others who may be present

● ● ● ●

Heal Your Emotions, Heal Your World

Once you realise what's holding you back, it's time to make changes in your life. Start with those closest to you, usually family members. If you're caught in unhappy family situations that seem to have no solution, you're not alone. Many families live in a state of hostility for years. Make no mistake, it's usually fear that keeps you from resolving family issues. Fear of taking the uncomfortable steps needed to repair love gone wrong lowers your vibrational ratio and may even trigger illness. It's important to smooth out the problems.

We are connected in many ways to our family members. They know exactly which buttons to push and if enough pushing goes on, your home may resemble a battleground. Your heart may hurt, quite literally, especially if your children are acting out. Until those in conflict accept the message of unconditional love, unhappiness will prevail.

Lack of communication presents a big hurdle. If your child has gone astray in his or her exploratory teen years, try your best to keep the conversational door open and the flame of love burning. If you have put in the groundwork during the first seven years of their lives, more often than not they'll return like moths to a flame.

I suggest that the member who is the most spiritually evolved be the one to do most of the work of forgiving. You may have to swallow your pride to take that first step toward mending the rift. Just do it. Bend over backward if need be. Doing everything in your power is worthwhile as a great depth of feeling may come from it. Sometimes, the simplest act of love can begin the process of mending a rift. If it can't be mended face to face, you can start the process by picking up the phone, sending a card or letter of love, or having flowers delivered. Be open about how much your loved one means to you. Small gestures can open the door to relationship repair.

When you forgive you must forgive from the depth of your heart. Shallow words will not reach your loved ones. You may have to try and try again, learning from previous awkward attempts along the way. Don't give up. When love is healed you'll feel incredible joy, signifying that your heart generator is working powerfully again. This means everything for your health and well being.

Another way to repair a love relationship is to just step aside for a while, giving emotions time to settle down. You can do this ever so nicely, be it with friends or with family members. This is a good way to handle things if you realise you're being used as a dumpee. If someone is using you as a target for their negativity, it can literally weaken your energy field. Get out of the way. There is a huge difference in talking things through in an adult manner and sheer negative dumping. Most dumpers don't want to work on themselves because they are not ready. Try to talk honestly with them to help them realise that when they are dumping, they are not taking ownership of their own issues. Once a problem like this is resolved, you will feel free, as though a huge weight has been lifted. Cleaning up your act literally cleans up your field.

Touch is vitally important to our well being, but sadly, the majority of humans are afraid to hug. It's quite amazing how many can't let their heart exude energy during a hug; you actually feel their body become stiff. Do yourself a favour and be relaxed during a hug to receive full benefit from the surge of positive energy coming your way. Exercise your good judgment if a person you want to hug seems reluctant. There may be a good reason. Ask first whether you can give them a hug.

Hugs can even improve your physical health. Dr David Bressler, director of the pain control unit at UCLA, recommends bear hugs as often as possible. "I often tell my patients to use hugging as part of their treatment of pain." Hugging has also been shown to lift depression, protect against illness, and stimulate the immune system. In Texas, Dr Robert Ryerson, chairman of the psychiatry department at Scott & White Clinic says, "Researchers discovered that when a person is touched, the amount of hemoglobin in their blood increases significantly. An increase in hemoglobin tones up the body, helps prevent disease and speeds recovery from illness."

Thoughts and feelings are connected to every part of our bodies. It's important for you to know why certain parts are suffering. I compiled the following list with Dr Jennifer Hunter, a holistic physician from Australia. We found it fascinating that our findings are closely related to texts from traditional Chinese medicine, some more than a thousand years old. We hope these explanations help you to connect your emotions needing work to body parts needing healing.

PITUITARY: Communication and control, remembers the pattern of all the emotional experiences of the person as a child before 7 years of age.

IMMUNE MOLECULE: Standing tall and leading the troops (i.e. the immune system) to victory and pride. Opposite is crumbling and giving up.

BALANCE SYSTEM: Harmony, able to weigh up all points of view and make sense. Opposite is confusion, feeling "out of sorts" and uncoordinated, going around in circles.

SINUSES: Self-judgment and acceptance: if positive the person will move forward with their life; if negative they become blocked and stuck.

TONGUE: Expression of sweet and happy feelings. Opposite is spitting out/speaking poisonous and vindictive feelings.

TEETH: Each tooth is energetically linked to a specific organ and therefore reflects the emotions as they correspond to that organ (see chart on page 86).

THYROID: Difficulty protecting their own energy

reserves due to poor communication with self and others. Tendency to ignore their own needs and to martyr themselves, to be unrealistic about how much work they can manage. They then feel burned out and crash emotionally and energetically.

LYMPHATICS: Not going with the flow, emotional blockages, not communicating their emotions to the self (self not communicating).

BRONCHIOLES & LUNGS: Feeling vital, alive and optimistic. The opposite is pessimistic and giving up (deflation is the negative emotion).

HEART: Feeling strong and powerful, happy and joyous. The opposite is a broken heart, a heart that no longer sings. Emotionally it wants to connect with the energy of music and rhythm/dance. (It naturally vibrates rhythmically.)

LIVER: Idealistic, sets very high standards with great vision for the future. It is very vulnerable to bitterness, anger and resentment — particularly if people or situations let them down or don't proceed according to plan. A healthy liver finds it easy to be flexible and accepts that their standards are different from others. In that way it doesn't get overheated nor become tissue-tight, which prevents its production of bile.

GALLBLADDER: Emotional triggers are often linked to parental issues. May have difficulty "going with the flow" of other people's plans. It likes to keep everything in order according to it's own set of rules and protocols — like a public servant. Alternatively, it can be too relaxed and easy going, never making plans to do anything.

DUODENAL/SMALL INTESTINE: Thinking, thinking, thinking. It is always processing, digesting and absorbing information. It reflects a person's strength of mind and intellect. But if they try to solve everything intellectually and logically they easily become stuck and anxious. (These emotions relate to the stomach.)

STOMACH: Easy for it to get worried and ruminate over little things. It can get greedy and want everything, much to its own detriment. Or the opposite and deny itself any of the luxuries of life. (This holding area relates its feelings to the pancreas, small intestine, liver and gallbladder).

PANCREAS: Satisfaction and contentment. It is very sensitive to all emotions. It is very sweet and loves to nurture and mother others. It can get very needy, particularly wanting others to nurture it.

SPLEEN: Very touchy and sensitive to feeling criticised by others. Can hold onto emotional upsets and grievances and then let them out in a big gush of emotions, often with little sensitivity to others. Like the pancreas, it also needs lots of nurturing, but may refuse the help when it is offered. (Often will reject regeneration, saying, "No I can do it myself".)

ADRENALS & KIDNEYS: Willpower and the will to

live. They can be easily frightened and fearful of the future (including the fear of death). This makes them susceptible to becoming workaholics and stressed out or burning the candle at both ends.

BLADDER: Self-confidence and feeling secure. It can get nervous, uptight and confused. There are often mixed messages about what's important (e.g. a busy person often puts off urination because there are more important things to do like working and making money). In turn, this affects the natural timing and flow.

MALE REPRODUCTIVE SYSTEM: Assertiveness and taking control over reproduction (this should not be confused with suppressing ejaculation). This is a complex subject because male and female sexuality is in a state of flux in our society. It is therefore no surprise that prostate cancer is on the rise. Interestingly it rarely kills, suggesting that men are trying to deal with the emotional challenges.

FEMALE REPRODUCTIVE SYSTEM: Receptive and feeling "clucky". Cancers of the female reproductive system are the most common, again reflecting emotional issues with sexuality and female roles in society.

COLON/LARGE INTESTINE: Making judgments and choices. Can get stuck or bogged down. Combine this with a toxic liver and the person may be too judgmental with themselves or others. Finding it difficult to let go or forgive and forget. This is a trigger for depression.

HIPS/PELVIS: Foundations of sense of self. Feeling

confident about who you are and what you do. Easily affected by the opinions of others and not feeling good enough or liked by others.

SPINE: Emotional burdens and memories. There are many charts that correlate different vertebrae to specific organs and emotions (just like the ones for the teeth).

NECK/CERVICAL: Doing tasks, activities, spending time with people when you don't really want to, but unable to communicate this until it's too late. Connected to emotions of the small intestine and thyroid.

UPPER THORACIC: Carrying a load that is too heavy. This can lead to a closing down, poor communication, giving up or lack of joy. Connection to the emotions of the lungs and heart.

LOWER THORACIC: Right side is connected to the emotions of the liver and gallbladder — anger and frustration. Left side is connected to the emotions of the stomach — appetite for life, greed and worry — and lymphatic system, going with the flow.

UPPER LUMBAR: Working and martyrdom. Connected to emotions of spleen and pancreas — sensitivity, nurturing, need and adrenals and kidneys — working; large intestine — holding on/letting go; and bladder — security, sense of self.

SACRUM: the foundation of the person and how they support themselves. So it relates to the emotions of the bladder and spleen. It is strongly influenced by the emotions of the hips.

SKELETAL SYSTEM: Affected by your emotional state. If these areas are showing weakness, it may indicate that you are blocking certain actions or feelings:

KNEES: You may want to kick out in anger.

ANKLES: You may fear taking the next step in your life.

SHOULDERS: You may be carrying the burden of another person's problems.

ELBOW: You may be trying to force someone to get out of your way or out of your life.

WRISTS: You may need to stop. You've had enough.

HANDS: You feel you are doing too much hard work.

• • • •

As our teeth are related to our emotions, the following chart will explain why you may be having dental problems. I suggest that you seek out a holistic dentist in your area to at least remove amalgam fillings to stop mercury from escaping into your body.

TOOTH CHART

UPPER RIGHT

11 and 12	Sinus – Ear – Tonsil
13	Sinus – Hips – Tonsil – Eye – Knee
14 and 15	Sinus – Nose
16 and 17	Sinus – Larynx
18	Duodenum – Middle Ear – Shoulder – Elbow – Circulation

UPPER LEFT

21 and 22	Tonsils – Sinus – Ear
23	Hip – Tonsil – Sinus – Eye – Knee
24 and 25	Bronchial – Sinus – Nose
26 and 27	Larynx – Sinus
28	Tetunum – Middle Ear – Shoulder – Elbow – Circulation

LOWER RIGHT

41 and 42	Ear – Sinus – Kidney – Bladder
43	Hip – Eye – Spleen – Tonsil – Liver
44 and 45	Breast – Larynx – Pancreas – Stomach
46 and 47	Nose – Bronchus – Thyroid – Lung
48	Shoulder – Elbow – Middle Ear – Heart – Small Intestine – Circulation

LOWER LEFT

31 and 32	Ear – Sinus – Tonsil – Kidney – Bladder
33	Hip – Eye – Knee – Tonsil – Liver
34 and 35	Breast – Larynx – Spleen – Stomach
36 and 37	Nose – Sinus – Lung – Large Intestine
38	Middle Ear – Shoulder – Elbow – Heart – Small Intestine – Circulation

UPPER RIGHT UPPER LEFT

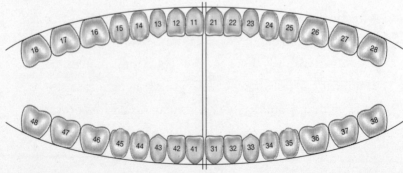

LOWER RIGHT LOWER LEFT

Emotional Dependency

Once awareness of childhood wounds and victimisation come to light, many people can release the emotional blocks they created. In the last several decades, psychologists and counsellors have been able to help many people get over limitations brought about by childhood trauma. Our DNA has evolved as well, helping us to recognise and remove these tangles of past un-discharged emotion from the computerisation, or memory bank, in our fields.

Sickness is a cloak of protection for people who believe that "as long as I'm sick I can get attention and sympathy." It can be used to control others as well. The roots of this poor-me syndrome may go back to childhood, when being sick was the only way to get loving attention from the parents. Or perhaps, the child was successful at avoiding school by reciting a list of symptoms. This gave them a sense of negative power.

Creative Chaos

We put so much effort into creating order in our lives, creating chaos can seem very threatening. Making changes necessitates giving up some old ways of being and creating new patterns of thought and behaviour. Unconscious, automatic actions may need to be brought to the surface and altered. Comfortable habits may need to be broken.

I'm always amazed at the misuse and mismanagement

of the body people become accustomed to. Habitual thoughts and actions may feel right because you're used to them (like sitting slouched in your chair), but they can be very wrong and harmful to your health. A period of perceived chaos and discomfort usually ensues when you begin to correct things.

The changes you make may be as challenging as finding a new job or as easily accomplished as adding an exercise regimen to your day. If your job is draining your energy, weakening your field, and threatening to make you ill, you really have no choice. Instead of focusing on the positives of leaving such a negative environment we concentrate on what could go wrong: will a new job be better, pay as much or more, a convenient commute? No wonder we tend to view change as a negative.

The interesting thing is that change creates a form of energetic panic in us, kicking us into high-energy mode where we find the power to achieve the necessary modifications. We feel a driving urge to get things back in order as quickly as possible. Scientists know that energy creates energy. How many times have you thought, "I can't do it, I don't have any energy, I feel too tired." But if you push yourself, you will become energised. Take action and before you know it, you'll find yourself climbing steps to higher levels.

My Emotional Freedom

Before the Christmas holiday, when I was about to start decorating my house, I had a devastating call from the owners telling me they had decided to sell the property. I could purchase it or leave when it was sold. A friend told me the house was probably up for sale because it was only fifteen feet from the cliff edge and land in the neighbourhood had started to slide. I was heartbroken. Insecurity set in big time. Where would I go? Where would I live now? My mind was racing.

I was walking in the woods trying to think when that deep inner thought interrupted my tears saying, "Robyn, don't cry, it's time to get out of the woods." Once again, God was the generator and I would be cared for. I needn't worry. But where would I go? For now, all I knew was that my dear son Aaron, who was working in television in London, had invited me to spend the millennium in that exciting city. I decided to stop dwelling on my negative feelings about losing the house and focus on the marvelous trip I was about to take.

New Dimensions in Healing

"Human beings and all living things are a
coalescence of energy in a field of energy
connected to every other thing in the world.
This pulsating energy field is the central engine
of our being and our consciousness."

Lynne McTaggart
The Field

Chapter Five
London for the Twenty-First Century

My sadness about leaving Olympia was offset by the
pleasure of travelling the globe once again. I spent
Christmas in Australia visiting my daughters and then met
my son, Aaron, in London where he was working in the
television industry. One of my friends from Australia was
staying in London too, trying to start a television station
dedicated to natural health. It was wonderful seeing her
again and she was very helpful in referring clients to me.
I began to plant some tentative roots.

I'd arrived in London with the manuscript for
Conversations with the Body, intending to send it to an agent
back in California who'd expressed interest in it. Then
Robert Holden, an author friend who admired my healing
work, sent the manuscript to his publisher. They sent me a
contract immediately and put it on the schedule for release
in February 2002. Knowing my book was to be published
in the UK provided impetus to stay. I asked a friend in
Seattle to hire a moving company to clear out the house
and put my furniture in storage. I could no longer put the

loss of my home out of my mind and I had to fight off sadness and negative feelings about it.

Living in a hotel seemed confining after having a house all to myself, but I adjusted quickly. Clients from around the UK came for sessions. Many from the States called for telephone sessions, and I was becoming more confident about being able to heal from a distance. To my delight, healing seemed even more successful by phone than in person, which I ascribe to the relaxation of my clients who no longer had to suit up and maneuver through traffic to show up at my door. They could stretch out comfortably on their own beds and easy chairs and go with the flow.

I was able to take time to explore London and visit sites of interest. Though it was prior to the 2001 attack on the World Trade Center, I felt a very intense inner warning that the London Underground held danger and promised myself not to travel on the tube train system. "Stay away," something was saying to me. And now, sadly, time has proved my inner guidance correct.

Aaron thought I was being paranoid. "Push through, Mum. Have a go. I'll come with you."

We took an escalator deep underground and I must admit I was impressed, especially when a very attractive red, white and blue train pulled in. We sat in a section where passengers faced one another. To our left was a pregnant woman, opposite her a man with his head buried in a newspaper. When we pulled into a station, the man got up and stood at the door to get off.

The pregnant woman called to him, "Excuse me, you left your parcel under the seat." She looked terrified.

"It's not mine," he muttered as he hit the platform nearly running.

The woman quickly jumped off the train and I followed at her heels. Aaron tried to reassure me that all was well, but by now I was on the platform and security guards were getting on the train. They gingerly grabbed the parcel and carried it away. Nothing my son could say convinced me to get back on. "Thanks for the ride but that's the last one," I said, and I meant it.

One unforgettable place I visited was the "Old Operating Theatre" in the bell tower of St. Thomas Church next to St. Thomas Hospital where Florence Nightingale once nursed. During the mid-1800s and early 1900s, doctors in top hats and tails with small white aprons covering their fronts performed amputations here in the tower where patients' screams could not be heard. Their patients were women from the hospital next door; most of the amputations were needed because limbs were badly infected. Surgery took place without anesthesia, which had not yet been developed.

Medical students and relatives of the patients sat in a tiered semicircular gallery to watch. Doctors worked with thick sawdust on the floor to catch the blood. To add to the grisliness, they had competitions to see who could amputate a leg the fastest while the gallery cheered. The record was just under a minute. A framed pen-and-ink sketch on the wall depicted a scene of four attendants holding the patient down while the doctor sawed away. People were smaller then, so the chairs and the operating table seemed made for youngsters, which compounded my revulsion. Sad letters were also displayed written by the women, who did not believe they would survive. One wrote, "If I don't die on the table from pain and shock, I will probably die from infection after."

As I viewed the operating theatre and exhibits, including barbaric surgical instruments, I felt the horror of it all as the negative frequencies engendered by those awful events were still implanted in the timber walls and furniture. Frequencies never go away. I had to work very hard to keep from taking in the negativity.

Doctors did not wash their hands before they operated nor did they sterilise instruments. They simply were totally ignorant that germs and bacteria existed until they actually saw them under microscopes. And now, just over a hundred years later, I can see germs without a microscope, my eyes closed and the client perhaps a thousand miles away.

I believe that I am the first wave of a new healing paradigm that others will be able to learn. But like nineteenth-century doctors who did not believe in germs before they could see them, the majority of people today cannot stretch their minds around the concept of natural energy healing — especially at a distance over the phone. They'd be very surprised to learn that healing is even more powerful when spoken directly into the ear. I keep letters from my many clients willing to go public with testimonials about their successful healings and post many on my web site. They are the proof of the pudding, so to speak. I love them for having the faith and trust to try this new method and for providing tangible proof that it works.

I had not been in London very long when foot-and-mouth, or mad cow disease broke out. Hundreds of cattle in the UK were diagnosed, while on the Continent, there were fewer. Europe injected their livestock; the United Kingdom slaughtered more than two million animals and burned their bodies in huge pyres that sent ominous clouds of dark smoke over the land. Though it may sound far-fetched, I actually felt the pain of the millions of animals put to death and I shed tears from the depth of my soul.

After nine dreadful weeks of slaughtering healthy animals along with those infected, substantially fewer animals were turning up with the disease. People wanted the killing stopped, but when would the right time come? Then miraculously in April 2001 a pure white calf was found alive under a pile of fifteen animals that had been dead for five days, including her mother. The farmer named her Phoenix and refused to put her down. The media picked up the story and Phoenix became a national hero, her face with its huge brown velvety eyes peering out from television and newspapers. Always sympathetic to the plight of animals, the British public cried out in one voice, "Let her live." Prime Minister Tony Blair finally called a halt to the slaughter.

I saw a very clear spiritual message in the events. Though most people missed it entirely, one archbishop interviewed on television believed, as I did, that the horror of the event was a spiritual cleansing for the country. There was the classical sacrificial lamb (cattle and sheep), the purification by fire, and the miracle birth of a pure white calf to put an end to the sacrifice. Since then, the level of consciousness has been rising in the United Kingdom, which had been energetically stuck in the past previously. Now I see more open-mindedness and a stronger movement toward spiritual awareness there.

My book came out on time and my publicist went to work. Every time I spoke with her on the phone, she was coughing. I wondered how she sounded to media people as she coughed her way through her explanations of my book. I agreed to heal her and was able to get rid of a virus that had been in the base of her lung for more than a year. She appreciated getting over her virus and arranged for a major newspaper to interview me. Their lengthy article about my work brought hundreds of enquiries from people seeking healing. There was no way I could see everyone on an individual basis, so I presented seminars in London, which proved very useful. The people were different from those I'd seen in the USA, however. The UK was definitely behind in enlightenment and alternative healing knowledge. It's catching up fast. Prompted by more illness and disappointment with the socialised medical system, the natural approach appeals to more and more people there.

Americans are much easier to work with as so many of them have an attitude of faith. In general, those with faith have bodies that are more pliable, their tissues are softer. It's apparent that their belief in Divine energy makes the difference. They tend to believe in God or at least in a higher power. For many, the category "spiritual but not religious" fits.

Some people are afraid that if they say the word God, they'll be seen as some kind of religious nutcase. These unfortunate people find it hard to love. God is love, after all, and clearly a threat to their pseudo-sophistication.

In my youth, we were taught that God was a man sitting up there in heaven looking down and judging us. I've certainly moved on, as have many others. I now realise that God is Divine, positive energy, a powerful generator connected to our heart generators. The generators are supposed to work in unison. When that occurs, when we resonate with spirit, we become powerful, healthy, creative and strong, filled with love and compassion. I'm not afraid to say "God bless you", not afraid to love and feel love.

Aaron called one day, all excited. "Mum, I'm now to be

based in London permanently." He'd landed a very good job with a major TV network. He went on, "Why not let me get you out of this hotel situation? Perhaps we can find a large apartment to share." I loved the idea and we went out to look.

We tried several real estate agents to no avail and were ready to give up for the day when I remembered another I'd seen across town. But this agent had nothing suitable either. We were dejectedly headed for the door when she sang out, "Wait a minute, I just remembered clients who own a spacious apartment. They're considering having the right people housesit and pay minimal rent."

The apartment was certainly everything she said, and the wealthy owners agreed to let us move into their beautifully furnished place at a very advantageous rate. And so my suitcases moved up in the world. God was pulling strings again. After eight years of travelling alone, it was superb to be with family once more.

I made the decision to attempt all work by phone, not that I was performing many healings at that point as my administrative work had become overwhelming since my book was published. Just answering daily emails took hours. I finally gave up on the computer as my sensitivity to electromagnetic frequencies (EMF) was becoming more acute. I found a person to print out emails, deliver them to me and send out my answers, which freed quite a lot of time for me to work on myself and heal others.

Going through my mail one morning, I came across a very distressing plea: "I have narcolepsy and I fell asleep at the wheel with my children in the car. Now I'm sleeping nearly all day and cannot get the children to school. Their education is suffering. Can you please help me?"

My heart went out to Kathryn Quinn, a 37-year-old medical secretary. Her case was rather complex. Her physician had diagnosed her as a borderline diabetic years earlier. He'd referred her to a neurologist when he learned of her inordinate need for sleep. The neurologist confirmed the diagnosis of narcolepsy and prescribed a narcolepsy drug, which worked like an amphetamine and was just as addictive. Quickly Kathryn graduated to taking six to eight pills a day to stay awake. As much as she wanted to quit taking them, she fell asleep and could not function without them. She had two young children and a partner who'd been seriously injured in an accident and remained unwell for two years. The drain on her energy was enormous and she became very depressed. Though she tried to keep her spirits up, her doctor eventually put her on an anti-depressant.

In addition to depression, narcolepsy and a diabetic condition, Kathryn also had a lesion on her face diagnosed by a dermatologist as basal cell carcinoma. Later she was to tear a cartilage in her knee while at the gym, which would, according to her doctor, require keyhole or arthroscopic surgery and weeks of therapy to repair.

I thoroughly enjoyed working with Kathryn. She really loved her life and wanted to be well enough to enjoy it. She was highly motivated and eager to follow my instructions to the letter. She had sessions with me by phone. Soon she was able to stop taking the anti-depressant and eventually cut down and finally stopped taking the narcolepsy drug, suffering no side effects. One must bear in mind that any chemical has to be stopped gradually. The quality of her life changed enormously, and she became a working mother who could actually cope with everything in her busy life. Her relationship with her partner improved, her children benefited, her job became easier. The tumour on her face receded and the cartilage in her knee was repaired to the extent that she could run again.

Kathryn sent me a long, touching letter of thanks. Her eagerness to be well certainly helped the healing process, but still, I expended a lot of energy diagnosing and healing her.

I'd been working so hard, I decided I needed some retail therapy. I'd seen some lovely shoes in a shop window and set off to try them on. They were a perfect fit and looked great. I slung the shop bag over my shoulder and crossed the road heading for the supermarket. Then I saw her: dirty, bedraggled, matted hair. My eyes dropped to her feet, which were covered in thick layers of newspaper tied on with string. My heart sank. Guilty thoughts raced through my head. I'd just spent a pretty penny on unnecessary shoes while this poor woman went without. A feeling of numbness swept over me. I dove into my purse and pulled out a twenty-pound note. She was rumbling through the rubbish dumpster by then. Ignoring the money I proffered, she pulled back her arm like a prizefighter and let me have a punch in my stomach that took my breath away. She followed with another blow to my arm.

I turned away still clutching the money, which she had not taken. My head reeled. Why? What was the message? I was only trying to help her. Obviously she was mentally unstable, evidenced by her garbled nonsensical yelling that haunted me for days. I was thankful that my working out had given me muscles that tightened automatically on impact or she might have caused real damage.

When I arrived back home, tears flowed behind my closed doors. I thought it through. What was the lesson? I've often given to street people since my days in Seattle where there were many of them. Every time I look at them I say a prayer for them realising that "there but for the grace of God go I." Homeless people are everywhere now, as few governments provide institutions to house them. I made up my mind not to give them money any more. My lesson was, Robyn, you can't help everyone. It's not possible to be all things to all people.

Of course, I've broken my rule since then but I'm careful to give to those who thank me with smiles, not fists.

I continued my healing work in London with excellent

results. Another client came along who touched me deeply. She was Sue Bracknell, a woman with a huge heart always full of love and caring for others. She had spent an extraordinary amount of money on trying to get well and nothing had worked. Friends in England have told me that getting well can cost at least 40 thousand pounds sterling, excluding airfare for treatment in various European clinics.

Sue had been to the finest Harley Street specialist, one of the most prominent in London, trying to get an accurate diagnosis concerning a mass in her neck. Over the course of nine years, she'd also tried chiropractic, Chinese medicine, reflexology, Indian head massage, acupuncture, cranial sacral therapy, physiotherapy, and a healer who charged in fifteen-minute increments.

Not one of these practitioners had found the huge haematoma I discovered in her neck. Sue's healing was very interesting. After eight sessions, the haematoma started to deflate like a balloon. During this process, masses of infection drained from the area as high as her ear, leaving a large hollow in her neck. Today, her neck has evened out and looks quite normal.

After her healing, she called to say that sunflowers had grown from seeds scattered near the guinea-pig pen outside her second storey bedroom window. They grew to gigantic heights, one to 17 feet tall. She had been playing my CD constantly and swore that its high vibration had been responsible for the extraordinary growth. Her local newspapers took photos of Sue with her giants and splashed them all over their pages. Of course Sue had no trouble winning the largest flower competition. Her only problem was propping them up and supporting the massive heads. Seeds sown the next year from the giants had stalks like tree trunks, she told me. We thought that size and strength would continue; however in the third year, they started to dwindle. Sue's health now did not need the CD, so its vibration no longer reached the sunflowers.

I hope to do some research in using my vibration for agriculture. In the 1960s, a Canadian biologist, Dr Bernard Grad of McGill University, Montreal, soaked seeds in two containers of salt water, one of which was given to a healer to lay hands on. Then he planted all the seeds. The seeds from the container held by the healer grew taller than the other batch. It's well-documented, provocative work I'd like to follow up. Plants and animals keep evolving and instinctively reaching for high vibrations to improve their strength and health.

Humans are supposed to be more intelligent but many people have trouble with the very notion of vibrations. Persons in lower vibrational dimensions fear anything that threatens the status quo. By taking a close-minded viewpoint, they are attempting to create a mental barrier against anything that would bring change. Essentially, they disempower themselves.

Cynics seem terrified of my work and of me, not only because they don't understand but also because high vibrations are very bright, like white light. Because those in low vibratory levels live mainly in the dark, bright light frightens them.

Chapter Six

The Human Energy Field

Working with the energy field is one of the most meaningful things I do. All illness starts in the body from vibrational weakness caused by negative frequencies in the field. I do a great deal of diagnosis from anomalies in the energy field and achieve excellent results by repairing energy circuits there. It is distressing that so many people still find it hard to comprehend and reject the very idea that bodies have energy fields. Fortunately, science is beginning to acknowledge this more subtle form of healing as open-minded physicians and other researchers are devising experiments to measure the field.

The search for an accurate description of the field has been going on for thousands of years. In *Future Science*, John White and Stanley Krippner reported that the human energy field has been described in more than ninety-five cultures around the world. For example, sages in India taught students to move universal energy, or prana, through their bodies to purify and heal themselves. Their breathing technique is remarkably similar to the one I teach. In ancient China, masters taught Qigong, a method for maintaining health by controlling the vital energy of the body.

In the Western world, the energy field is depicted in paintings showing haloes of Divine energy around the heads of Christ and the saints, whose miraculous cures are well known. In the sixteenth century, a physician known as Paraclesus made the amazingly accurate observation that the vital force is not enclosed inside an individual but radiated within and around him like a luminous sphere, which could be made to act at a distance.

Since the beginning of the twentieth century, some instruments have been developed that can pick up emanations from the human energy field. Kirlian electrophotography, developed in the 1940s by Russian scientist Semyon Kirlian, allows us to see the energy "corona" around human beings as beautiful colours on the photographic plate. Many people refer to it as the Kirlian aura. In tests, patterns of light coming from a subject's fingertips offered diagnostic information about the presence of cancer and other diseases in the body. But even electrophotography cannot do justice to the glories of a healthy energy field, which vibrates with beautiful vivid colours and almost buzzes with high vibrations.

Valerie Hunt made use of telemetry equipment that had originally been developed so NASA could transmit recordings of astronauts' muscle and heart activity back to earth. In her laboratory at UCLA, she was able to measure changes in the energy field of subjects undergoing Rolfing (a deep tissue massage). In my opinion, her experiments described in her book *Infinite Mind* present the most definitive scientific proof that each one of us has a measurable energy field. It not only exists, but other people can affect it.

In recent experiments in China, researchers studied the possible effects of vital force, or Qi energy, on distant objects. The most amazing finding was that instruments in Beijing picked up Qi transmitted from a Qigong master in the United States. This 1993 study was important as it again verified my own finding that I could heal people thousands of miles away over the telephone. With evidence now mounting in scientific laboratories, I hope that increasing numbers of people will see the value of energy healing.

• • • •

One of my clients in Seattle had taught me a valuable lesson about energy. John had arrived on a rare sunny day and we'd sat on the balcony to get acquainted. His friend Fran remained inside the house looking worried. I could tell she really loved him. Even before John told me he'd been diagnosed with lung cancer, the frequency fluctuations in his energy field communicated to me that his lungs were in trouble. I also saw weak frequencies in his field in the area of his heart. I saw something else there too, but I wasn't sure yet what it was telling me.

During my scan of his lungs, I wasn't surprised to see damaged cells and tissue from long-term cigarette smoking. There was no doubt in my mind that smoking had caused his cancer.

"I hope you have stopped," I said.

"No." he answered. "Since Gloria died two years ago, I guess I smoke even more. We were married for forty years. I still miss her."

"But John," I said in desperation, "don't you understand that every puff feeds the cancer? If you want to become well, you will have to stop." And then I knew what else I was picking up from his energy field. For the first time since I'd been healing people, I was faced with a client who wanted to die.

My affiliation with the ministry of spiritual healers had helped make me comfortable talking about death. I'd learned that some people almost need permission to leave even though they know deep down that it's time. When I entered John's energy field on his next visit, I was expecting it to have begun showing clarity but instead I saw that it was time for him to return home to be with his long-term partner. Deep down in his heart and pituitary gland I could see darkness. He was unable to put aside his overwhelming grief. It was constantly with him.

I asked him gently, "Are you sure you do not want to join Gloria?" He became very quiet for a moment. "No, I don't think so", he said. I continued with his session but had an overwhelming feeling of despair, knowing that it was his time to go.

When he arrived for his third session, I noticed that his demeanour had changed. He seemed somehow lighter and freer. "Robyn, you were so right, I just had trouble coming to grips with it." He cried for a minute then went into a deep altered state. There he sat with the late afternoon sun shining on his bowed head, eyes closed, his lips in a gentle smile, almost as if he were home with Gloria already.

John's friend Fran was waiting in the next room hoping to hear that I could miraculously make her beloved friend well. When I told her that he wanted to be with Gloria, she wept uncontrollably. Three weeks later she called to tell me of John's peaceful passing. She added that he smoked right to the end.

I felt that I had passed a huge milestone being able to speak about death. People know, at some level, when their time has come. It shows up in their energy fields as snow of varying colour, from gray to black. It's different from negative energy, as death is simply the next step in our journey.

I don't think that ordained religious ministers at deathbeds realise fully what they are achieving by clearing negative energy for the dying person's return home. I had intuitively known I should build up enough positive power in John's field to help boost him through several spiritual dimensions on his way home to his beloved Gloria in heaven.

Another married couple I worked with went in a very different direction, building positive energy as a team and bringing their vibrations into harmony. Gail had been in bad health since 1974 suffering from Lupus, Hepatitis A and B, and lacking energy. She had been growing progressively worse and her heart was close to failing. Her husband, Tom, was very depressed, couldn't sleep, had impaired vision and terrible pains in his legs and stomach. He was skeptical when Gail started working with me, doubting that healing could be done on the phone but as Gail's condition improved, he asked me for healing too.

Gail and Tom worked on keeping their relationship positive and encouraged each other to follow my directions. One would say to the other, "Have you done all your breathing today?" I was thrilled to see them enhancing each other's healing process. Gail wrote, "After thirty years, I finally have my life back. I'm happy, healthy, and confident and can finally create my dreams." And Tom's note was equally positive: "I have new clarity of mind which allows me to face all that life puts before me with a strong body and a zest for life." (Their letters are on my web site in their entirety.) It's a wonderful feeling for me to witness the strength that continues to come into their lives. Their collective energy is so positive, anything is possible.

Positive Energy Fields

By now, seeing energy fields had become second nature to

me. All things have an energy field, even rocks. Everything on the planet is connected by Divine God energy. This is the energy that is drawn in by neurons inside the fontanel area. It circulates through our bodies and out through our energy fields. It is originally pure positive energy and if we keep it that way, we'll be healthy. The easier the birth, the more aligned they are. If a person had a breech or forceps birth, these neurons end up out of alignment, not in the correct place. During every session, my first protocol is to align those neurons.

At birth the colour of the human energy field is pink. This develops into a range of nine beautiful colours with maturity: dark blue on the bottom, yellow, orange, green, red at elbow height, light blue, violet, cream, with Divine white light at the top. The crystal white Divine colour hovers above and around our heads. This is the halo, which is larger and brighter on people who work hard to have a strong positive field.

In my view, energy constantly enters through the top of the crown, where it is magnetised by the band of neurons situated in front of the fontanel. It collects in our forehead, the holding area. We have two choices of what to do with this energy. We can use it to create positive or negative vibrations. We renew this decision every minute of every day as we decide what to think, how to feel, how to act and respond, what to do. Our thoughts, attitudes and actions are always under our control. It may take a considerable effort to master them, as the body will only tolerate one energy at a time, positive or negative.

The Heart Generator

Positive energy has a far higher frequency than negative and functions in a very different way. Spiraling down from the top of the head, it is channelled through the heart where it is charged with the feeling of love. No one can truly know anything unless they've felt it and only the heart can produce the love energy needed.

We now know that the heart is not just a pump house for our blood. It is also a powerful electrical generator capable of recharging itself and the energy it circulates with positive force. The supercharged energy keeps moving, exiting from the bottom of the heart as the frequency of love. ("I love you from the bottom of my heart" is literally true.) From there it cycles inside our bodies in a clockwise direction, feeding our body parts along the way. Still powerfully positive, it then exits through our pores to feed our circuits in the field. A field charged with love exudes joy.

When you feel warmth in your heart region, your generator is working. A loving relationship can stimulate it, but you can activate it in other ways. A beloved pet can help or anything else you hold dear. If you love music, listen to as much as you can. Our energy field can be likened to the harmonious flow of a colourful orchestra playing nothing but positive melodies.

Negativity in the Energy Field

If a person is in a negative state of mind, I see negativity exiting on both sides of the head just in front of the temples. As it merges with the field, negativity wreaks havoc with the circuits, unless counteracted with positive affirmations within twenty seconds. It knows exactly where to lodge in the weakest circuits, lowering their vibrations. It becomes destructive; the person wants to destroy. Lower frequencies can and usually do lead to body breakdown. This occurs because negative energy, three times more powerful than positive, builds explosive power that always has to erupt in anger or other form of hostility. Once laden with negativity, circuits try to clear themselves by exploding into the body to create illness. Afflicted circuits can only cause us harm. There is no up side.

Negative energy is denser than positive energy. The higher the frequency, the less dense or subtler the matter. Floating side-by-side in a pool, a person with high positive vibrations can easily float, but a negative person would tend to sink. You can apply the same principle to their lives in general. Negative people have trouble staying afloat in every way. In fact, people often refer to feeling heavy when they're ill. I strive to stay out of their low vibrations and raise them to my high vibration where love, health and happiness exist.

As time goes on, I detect and identify more negative

frequencies from common stresses in our personal environments: cleaning products, chemicals in our food, microwave ovens, computers and other electronic equipment that every household owns.

Lately I've begun to see "fusions" in the field, jam-ups of a group of frequencies. Mobile phones are the culprits most of the time, but electric shock can create fusion as well. So can old frequencies left in a place by highly charged negative incidents in the past. Jammed energy stops the flow and growth of the field.

It doesn't matter whether you send or receive calls on your mobile, the damage is done either way. Landlines are fairly benign in terms of electrical pollution and fax machines are reasonably mild as well. But recently I realised I was energetically clearing phone line connections between my clients and myself.

If you are a city dweller, you probably have to deal with pollution and massive electromagnetic (EMF) problems. Beware of commercial industry going on in your area. Inhalation of poisonous waste can, after a period of time, affect every cell in your body. Not until recently did human beings walk under power lines nor cope with frequencies from a wide range of electronic products. Certainly we're adaptable, but people's lives have been "improved" so rapidly, we hardly use anything that was commonplace fifty years ago. We have computers, computerised appliances — an endless number of household gadgets pulling electrical power into our homes, and more are invented every day. I remember my father telling me that when TV was introduced a warning was printed at the bottom: "Sit at least eight feet from this set to avoid radiation." Now mothers plunk their babies and small children directly under it; there are no warning signs on today's sets. Do they think that after only 50 years of evolution our systems are magically going to cope with it?

Manmade electricity runs counterclockwise through our systems. But God energy runs clockwise. We're basically going against nature, and we are now seeing the consequences.

A field with interference from negative frequencies is something like a radio dial that is not exactly on the station. You become tense and frustrated trying to listen, your thoughts become jumbled, and you may have pains in your head. You may experience the same problems if your energy field is not clear of negative frequencies.

When it is clean and running on positive energy you will come out of the haze and experience clarity in all areas of your life. Wellness, joy and love follow and you become attuned to a higher frequency zone where all things are possible.

All body parts are purely positive. They become negative from invasions of disease, parasitic infection, bacteria and other conditions. Even genetic weakness has to be triggered into action by negative energy in the field. People born with disabilities are working with karma brought in from other lifetimes or have chosen a lifetime of complications to boost others.

Every person has certain genetic weaknesses, although they usually don't bother us until weakened circuitry in the field gives them a chance to manifest in the body. For example, you might have the recurring thought, "My mother and father had a certain disease, and maybe I will get it." Now all you need in your life is something as simple as a relationship heartache to weaken your energy circuits and trouble is on the way. Every thought is powerful electrical energy that triggers any body weakness and does its worst to create a self-fulfilling prophecy.

Negativity in the field looks like television snow. It is dull and stagnant, lacking flow and movement, with no apparent colour. As the healing progresses, colour begins to surface but not until the negativity is cleansed and the field starts to blossom. I get enormous joy watching vibrant colour return. It's like turning up a dimmer switch on a lamp. The field moves and flows, enhanced with glowing colours far prettier than a rainbow. Sometimes, a person restored to radiant health has a field so bright I cannot see the state of their circuits. It glows me out.

If I must cleanse the field every session and strengthen the client's will to be positive, progress will be slow even though I'm strengthening the body biologically. A proactive client who works with me in a team effort exhibits exciting changes in feelings and attitudes. One way I can tell when healing takes a turn for the better is by a change in the vibrational tone of the client's voice. It becomes stronger and clearer. The wounded inner child disappears.

If clients continue to help me, healing will be super successful. They become captains of their ships and their fields expand in volume, becoming rich with colour and radiance. A field in this condition needs little or no help. It never ceases to amaze me how different it can look after being dark and sluggish laden with negative interference.

To remove the darkness, I strongly focus my energy tool against it, holding the focus with a powerful concentrated effort. The darker and more severe the negativity in the field, the longer and stronger I must work. Depending on the severity of negative frequencies, I apply huge effort to lift them. Usually they lift off little by little and appear to float away.

A cautionary note: many people have difficulty learning how to balance the large volume of energy coming from their field as they become well. This newfound energy can lend power to the memories of lost days when they were ailing and they find themselves burning out. When the power in the field declines, the body may, after the illness subsides, reproduce ailments suffered during the illness because it has memory. This occurs because it's not being fed constant positive energy from the field. However, the discomfort from the pre-existing ailment is different and goes away when field energy is restored, usually from sleep and rest. This can be likened to a rundown flashlight battery that emits a beam that's much weaker than one with a fully charged battery.

After a turn from illness into the wellness zone, newfound energy wants to surge. It wants to fly, to leave the body if it could. There's a real danger you'll overdo it and crash into a healing crisis. Then comes oppression and extreme tiredness with pain coming in, feeling the way it felt when your vibration was down.

Grounding Pole

When you feel your energy soaring too fast you can do the following exercise to give yourself a good level day, day after day, rather than going through exhausting ups and downs.

Imagine a horizontal pole above your head, at least as large as a broomstick.

Every time your energy wants to soar, imagine yourself grasping the pole as hard as you can.

Come back to the pole again and again.

● ● ● ●

Each of us has a computerised version of every moment of our entire life as part of our energy field. Clairvoyants are able to act like search engines, searching millions of bits of information about us and our spiritual connections to the deceased and to people in our lives, past and present. This is how psychics access our past, present, and future lives. Every bit of information is stored in each person's field, and some talented readers can call up anything they want to know about a person faster than the speed of light. Pictures or words show up as if they were on a computer screen. The energy field's capacity to store and retrieve information is probably what earlier psychics like Edgar Cayce, who did such wonderful work before computers existed, referred to as the Akashic records.

When I need to know what's holding clients back from progressing with their healing, I sometimes find the information in their fields. Perhaps the person is still sad about things that occurred in her childhood or angry with her current boss. When I find the errant thoughts, I talk them through with the client, gently urging her to confront what's holding her back, either by herself or with a therapist. A combination of therapy and my mind control techniques will generally eliminate even the toughest problem. Sometimes problems will come up by themselves, and the client will tell me. During distance healing on the phone, I intuitively know I have to work on finding the obstructions in the field at that time.

Maintaining a Positive Energy Field

Know that the mind can either take you to heaven or dump you in hell. Every time you have a negative thought or feeling, you need to disempower it, especially matters concerning the past, or something or someone that's pushed your buttons. Deal with these matters as quickly as possible to prevent field circuit damage. We all need daily work on ourselves to ride herd on fear, anger, jealousy, lust, deceit, guilt, depression, shame and every other sneaky feeling that may creep in if you're not vigilant. I can promise you that staying in the higher frequency range and playing in God's playground is worth far more than the effort you'll expend to get there. I'm forever encouraging myself inwardly.

The first line of defence against incipient negativity is my easy four-step Breath of Life technique. Use it within twenty seconds of the time negativity enters your mental, emotional, physical, or spiritual space.

• • • •

Breath of Life

Take a deep breath through the nostrils

Hold it for a count of eight while repeating a positive affirmation to counter negativity.

While holding your breath, visualise yourself doing something active like running on a beach

Blow out the negative thoughts through pursed lips, releasing them to the cosmos, directing them to the sun for purification.

Repeat eight times.

This simple method is actually a powerful technique of

mind mastery. Besides clearing negativity, remembering to use it means you're becoming more self-aware and self-disciplined every day. Self-confidence and personal development are not far behind.

Another simple technique is to start your day by opening your eyes every morning and saying, "Today I'm going to have a totally positive day." I'm not certain that anyone has ever had a day without the tiniest bit of doubt or negativity creeping in, but it's a worthy goal. When you begin this practice, your mind usually jumps in before your feet hit the floor. Until it's trained, the mind will never allow you to be free.

Start by taking the Breath of Life several times a day. Set aside specific times, just to develop self-discipline. Do a certain number of repetitions, at least eight, and more if you can do so comfortably. Allow this easy practice to become established in your schedule. You'll find additional suggestions for mind training in Chapter 12, Accessing Higher Dimensions.

Though it may seem a daunting task to reprogram your mind and keep your energy field clean, you'll find it easier day by day. If you remember to practice, your rewards will be great. Not only can you achieve and maintain a reliable state of glowing health, but you can also help make the world a better place. By becoming aware and evolved enough, and holding a firm intention, we may well remove sickness and disease from the planet.

Chapter Seven
Embryos from the Heart

Getting pregnant is not as easy as it once was. Many women wait to start families in order to devote their younger, more fertile years to their careers. For them the delay may prove costly. If they wait too long, they may remain childless. But conception may prove to be a problem even for those who desire children in their prime childbearing years.

In Vitro Fertilisation clinics are busy and popular now, as woman after woman seeks help to conceive a child, having found it impossible on their own. In my opinion birth control pills are to blame for many of these cases. The pills keep a woman's body in a state of permanent pregnancy, which is completely unnatural. Since the early days when the pill came on the market, I've believed that the second generation of women whose mother used the pill would be the most severely impacted. With evidence mounting, I remain firm in that opinion. These pills were pushed by the medical profession with no testing or thought for future generations. Women who took them at their doctors' recommendations should never feel guilty.

I believe that the morning after pill is the better alternative for birth control, as it is kinder to the woman's body. This has been the topic of some ethical and moral debate, but in my view there is no problem. Life in the embryo as we know it begins with the first heartbeat, three and one-half to four weeks after conception. Prior to the first heartbeat, the energy is used to develop the heart's tissues. As the heart begins to beat, it gives a sort of kick-start to the baby's field and then the embryo becomes a person. You have to have the heartbeat to build the field.

Wonderful discoveries are being made to enhance conception, delivery, and the care of infants. Expectant mothers — and fathers — take classes in everything from warm-water birth to baby massage and mother-and-baby exercise classes. One interesting study revealed that premature babies who received massages grew 47 percent faster than their unmassaged peers.

In 2002, Cindy contacted me to help her hold onto a pregnancy implanted by a fertility clinic. She informed me that she'd never had a problem conceiving but had had a very difficult time holding onto her pregnancies beyond four weeks, the time when a baby's heart usually starts beating. So far, four embryos had spontaneously aborted.

I had not worked with embryos before but believed I knew what to do. "I will try to help," I told her. "Next time you conceive, call me at three weeks if you can."

Before long, the phone call came. "I'm at three weeks with this one," she said. During the first part of our phone session, I could see that Cindy's body was in very good condition with the exception of a weakness in her liver that showed up in her field. I quickly repaired it.

When I looked into Cindy's uterus to see her microdot embryo, I became quite concerned. I tiptoed in and discovered a tiny, very upset being who wanted nothing more than to leave. "Oh no," I thought, "how can I help it change its mind?" Not knowing what to do or how to treat it, I inundated the embryo with enormous surges of love energy, the most love I could muster from my reserves.

Next day, I saw the same thing. The baby seemed to want to leave. I repeated the love treatment and hoped for the best. I had to tell Cindy, preparing her for the worst. On the third day, for some reason I didn't quite understand, I tenderly roughed a small section of tissue in the uterine wall and ever so gently guided this tiny dot into what I considered to be a nest. I instinctively knew where, though its back was only a dot. Once again, I poured love into the tiny embryonic being. Next day it was much more relaxed and seemed to be at ease about its upcoming birth. Cindy needed to know about this.

"I think Baby is going to stay," I informed her.

"Oh Robyn, I hope so, I can't keep going through these losses."

Next day I knew Baby was going to stay and I told Cindy

we could take a break. Intuitively, I knew that Cindy was carrying a girl. She was thrilled when I told her. Two weeks later, I had an overwhelming urge to check in, as I could easily do from any distance. Good thing I had, as she was attached to the wall. Without saying anything to Cindy of my midnight visit, I freed her. You cannot imagine how frightened I was. My mind filled with questions. Will this baby be okay? Will it have a mark on her back where she had been attached to the wall of the uterus? I decided to wait before telling Cindy. She was going through an emotional period and her slightest upset might be too much for the unborn child, whose hold on life was tenuous at best. I can honesty say this was the only time I ever held back anything that occurred in session.

Throughout her pregnancy Cindy continued to ring me up for the occasional session. We rarely made appointments in advance. Approximately mid-term Cindy came down with a flu virus, which created fluid around Baby's heart. I was able to drain it out successfully. Six months into the pregnancy, I discovered that Baby had the umbilical cord around her neck. This would at least make the birth dangerous and could possibly choke her in utero. I would have to find a way to fix it. Working very quickly, I dissected it at the navel and disengaged it from her neck. The process went beautifully.

When Megan was born, Cindy rang to say that she was a beautiful bouncing baby. Now came the part I'd been dreading. I'd been carrying stress from the moment I'd freed the embryo from the uterine wall, worrying that I'd left a scar on her.

"Does she have any marks on her back?" I asked. I knew my voice was shaking.

Much to my relief, Cindy answered "No. She's perfect in every way." I then told her about the night I'd found the embryo attached to the wall and had been afraid I'd left a scar on her precious, pure baby in the process of freeing her. Cindy did not mind at all, she had exactly the baby she'd dreamed of.

Megan is now going on three and, her mom told me recently, is a very advanced soul. She has strong ESP abilities, possibly from working with me in the womb. The only problem is, she expects everyone to have powerful intuition and ESP.

One of the very interesting phenomenon was Megan's ability from the womb to get her mother to call me when she needed help. Many times Cindy called me on the spur of the moment. "Hi Robyn, I just thought I'd say hello and check in with you." She told me later that most of the times she'd called, she'd had no idea why she was prompted to pick up the phone. It had just "felt right."

I feel blessed to be able to see into the womb. My very favourite thing to observe is a baby sucking a thumb just as it would after birth. They're so adorable! I'd often thought I should have had more babies — well here they are. I feel like a Fairy Godmother.

Cindy had friends who were also trying for in vitro fertilisation, Kellie and Grant, who had built Cindy and her husband their lovely new home. When they learned of Megan's birth, they approached me to work with them as Kellie had recently carried a baby for five months before it spontaneously aborted. It had been a devastating experience for both of them.

That time, it had taken four tries for Kellie to get pregnant, so I gave her three preparation sessions and told her to call me when the next fertilised eggs were ready. The call came quickly. Two fertile eggs were about to be implanted in Kellie.

The day after implantation, I scanned the two tiny dots cautiously, making quite sure that my energy was entering the womb very gently. I was surprised to see what appeared to be bruising on one of the eggs. I somehow knew it to be a boy baby. I kept constant vigilance during the following week. One afternoon I saw blood and kept cleaning it away to see where it was coming from. There appeared to be a leak in his blood supply, which I repaired. At this point, he seemed to be struggling for his life. Two hours later he appeared to be more settled.

Two days later his colour was quite dark. My mind reeled. Had I lost him? No, there was still life. I told Kellie and Grant what I was finding after every visit. Working from a distance can be exhausting for me. The thoughts that go through my mind when I come upon unexpected findings I've never seen before amaze me. Why was he so dark? I had not met Kellie and Grant in person; perhaps one of them had an African bloodline. Or perhaps it was not their egg. Could the wrong one have been implanted?

I rang my physician friend, Jennifer Hunter in Australia to ask what I might be seeing. "Your first thought was correct," she said, "it's probably bruising. The eggs have to get handled so much." I was relieved to learn that I hadn't been seeing things that were not there.

I could do no more over the next two days as the embryo began to shrivel away. Examination at the clinic proved that he was lost. I was deeply saddened. I had worked so hard trying to keep him alive. This tiny bruised dot valiantly struggling to stay alive made me realise how powerful the fight for life can be. His week of life was not in vain. His message to the world was: You have life, make the most of it, honour and live it.

It was incredible to watch the speed of growth of the girl baby. The most important thing now was to get Kellie past the five months mark, to keep her vibration up. This was not easy as she and Grant were highly emotional at this time, having decided to bury the ashes of the baby they'd lost after five months of pregnancy in their garden.

As I mentioned, I know instinctively if there are problems needing immediate attention, and I can attend to them without personal connection with the client at the time. On one visit to Kellie, I discovered an infection in the womb. "Oh no!" I thought, "not now!" With embryos — or with anyone with serious brain damage — inflammation can create critical problems. I had to tell her that we were going to need a full session to get rid of it. Kellie decided to have a test just to make sure and the clinic verified the infection I had seen.

I certainly understand why Kellie and Grant or other new clients might find it hard to understand how I know what I know and seek verification from their doctors when I relate problems found during my work with them. After discussing the infection with their doctor, who wanted to put Kellie on a course of powerful antibiotics, they decided to stick with my work and not take the prescribed medication. I did not prompt them in any way; they simply followed their own intuition. I'm happy to report that all is well, their baby girl, Sally was born not only normal but also exquisitely beautiful. No surprise there. Every time I'd worked with Kellie I'd said, "She'll be so pretty."

These darling little embryos take me back, not only to my own babies, but also to the time I learned to knit when I was fifteen. I found a knitting pattern book in the store, showing page after page of pretty little baby booties. I decided to knit some and give them to neighbours who were pregnant. I didn't stop until I'd knitted a dozen delicate little pairs, filled them with soft white tissue, and packed them in white boxes. I was happy at how beautifully they turned out. Maybe this was therapy, part of my healing process from loss of my beautiful mother. Or perhaps they were seeds being sewn for my future healing mission.

Many children are enthusiastic and eager to work with me. It's as though they know this work by heart. Even as young as three years old, they love their sessions and want to call me on the phone by themselves. Because of the power of my work, I have to work very quickly with little ones. I am able to determine just how much they can take and for how long. It's theoretically possible that my work is too strong for children, but it's never been a problem in reality.

Beverly called me to ask me to help her son Bobby, who was not quite three years old. His young life had been a nightmare of surgeries, medication, tubes, shunts, and other apparatus — and worst of all, endless pain. From birth he had been very irritable and at six weeks, an ultrasound on his tiny head revealed serious hydrocephalus, which caused severe headaches.

The neurosurgeon diagnosed schizencephaly — abnormal formation of the ventricles in the brain — and said that there had been an interruption when the cells were migrating in utero. Bobby had to have surgery to place a ventricular shunt to drain cerebral spinal fluid into the abdomen. Six weeks later, the valve had to be replaced, requiring additional surgery. When he was six months old, it malfunctioned again causing subdural hematoma.

Another surgery ensued to install drains. Beverly was very frightened by his stressed condition when he came from the operating room. She could not hold Bobby nor move him from the position he was in for fear the drains would shift and cause serious damage.

Beverly very wisely wrote affirmations for Bobby and recorded them to play back to him frequently. A few months later, the neurosurgeon said that he could not understand why Bobby's hydrocephalus had corrected to the extent it had. By the age of two, all of Bobby's apparatus had been removed. He wanted it out of his body, as there was too much pain associated with it. By now, however, his eyesight had been disrupted, perhaps from too much surgery, and he suffered seizures that were very hard to control. Bobby was still irritable, feeding was difficult and his muscle tone had become rigid, causing his spine to curve. When he was two and a half, he had surgery to insert a feeding tube, but the site never healed correctly and was constantly infected.

Beverly found it extremely difficult to handle and position her little boy. She was getting burned out looking for answers and had almost no relationship left with Bobby's father or her other children. The entire family was in crisis.

This is when Beverly called me. I was booked solid and was also scheduled to go on a long trip so I sent her copies of *Conversations with the Body* and my CD, *Dimensional Healing*. I called her when I returned to learn that Bobby had listened to *Dimensional Healing* every night and it had calmed him enough so he could sleep. We proceeded to do several sessions with Bobby over a six-month period. He was still unable to eat and was coping with constant seizures and unbearable spinal pain. I worked to strengthen the malfunction in his brain. If I could achieve this, I could perhaps get the electrical current working. I succeeded in making a significant improvement, which brought about positive changes in his eyesight and diminishing of his seizures. I wanted this child to be able to eat and digest food normally and worked on his stomach to bring this about. His mother was thrilled when the day came for removal of the feeding tube, which we achieved using no surgery. I knew it was time and gave her directions for removing it. We then had to think about what to feed him. I planned a diet of bland food for the first week, gradually adding different items until he was able to eat normally.

Initially, I was appalled at the level of pain this child had endured in his short life. During every session, I took care of the places where he hurt, doing a great amount of work on his terribly contorted spine. I worked hard to achieve alignment by stretching out his spine and opening up space between his discs and vertebrae. He actually grew eighteen inches over a couple of months from my stretching of his body. He now sits in his wheelchair with no problem and can be taken out for long walks in the fresh air. His spine is far less rigid, so he can lie on his back to be massaged.

He loves this gentle rhythmic touch. Instead of whining constantly, he now giggles; his vision is improving to the extent that he can focus on people and certain pictures. He started to communicate more with those around him, much to everyone's delight. I'm truly thrilled that Bobby's devoted mother has some peace in her life now and time for the other members of her family.

Will he ever be a normal little boy? The important thing for Bobby is not to be measured to some standard but to live comfortably in a family that loves him and is holding steady around him. I was fortunate to meet Bobby; it's amazing how souls like his can accomplish so much in their own loving ways.

I have also had the privilege of working with many of the indigo children, as they are known. Born with special spiritual and psychic gifts, their major problem is the outdated, impersonal teaching methods they are exposed to. The ABCs are boring and frustrating for these advanced little souls. The oldest are now in their teens and sadly many have been labeled as troublemakers because they cannot concentrate on the rote schoolwork that they find simplistic and annoying.

Physicians seem to think it's fine to give them Ritalin and other neurological medications to flatten their exuberance, enabling teachers and parents to control them. How is a drug-numbed brain expected to process anything? The brain is a transformer that compiles information in the field. It needs to be allowed to do this delicate, important work without interference. Many indigo children are giving up and leaving, as suicide tendencies are among the dangers of psychoactive medications.

Waldorf Schools, based on Rudolph Steiner's teachings, are the best places to educate incredibly gifted indigo children. According to educator Joseph Chilton Pierce, author of *The Magical Child*, Waldorf education gives children a space where they know they belong and are welcomed, wanted, and safe — the ideal learning situation. To reinforce acceptance, "every teacher touches each student every day with a hand on the shoulder, a handshake, or hug, both as they come into school and as they leave... If there is no assurance of safety, the child must use a good portion of its energy in defence mechanisms, which divides the mind and splits attention."

Steiner speaks of the six-to-seven-year-old child "coming down fully" into the physical world and body. He insisted we should leave abstract learning until children are older. "If you honour the child's development stage, as Steiner insisted and Waldorf does, learning is a spontaneous, joyful, and happy experience. It is play."

Treated correctly, these evolved souls will work themselves into powerful positions in the world and bring about enlightened changes that humankind so desperately needs. Interestingly, most indigo children are males because the male genes lead the way for future evolution.

As children, they have an extraordinary need to be loved and touched lovingly, as much of the work they will do is with the vibrations of their hearts. This doesn't mean that you let them run wild. Every child grows into a better human being by being taught right from wrong. You have to love them, discipline them, and show them the way.

HeartMath Institute in northern California has been researching every aspect of the heart, as I have, but they use different modalities to search for answers. Their researchers have come up with scientific proof of the existence of a "little brain in the heart." The embryonic heart actually develops and begins to beat prior to the development of the brain.

I have always known that each person's program for this lifetime is located in the heart. It's important to follow your heart because it truly knows the plan. Besides knowing what you were put on this earth to do and be, the heart is the centre of the human attributes which help make dreams come true: wisdom, courage, compassion, strength, positive energy, and most important of all — love. Jesus did not speak of the heart as an electrical generator with its energy field containing circuits, but he did urge us to love one another. His simple teachings elevated the human race. His message of love was more evolved by 3000 years than the states of mind prevalent when he lived.

Researchers at HeartMath are demonstrating that "the messages the heart sends the brain not only affect physiological regulation, but can also profoundly influence perception, emotions, behaviours, performance, and health."

They work with people of all ages and have developed programs that help everyone, from business executives to schoolchildren, create positive emotional states. Such information might be helpful for expectant mothers as well. HearthMath research "has shown that our heart's field changes distinctly as we experience different emotions, is registered by the brains of people around us, and also appears to be capable of affecting cells, water, and DNA studied in vitro."

Women through the ages have showered love on their unborn children, have sung to them, whispered encouraging words to them, and in general have recognised that they are truly communicating with them in the womb. I'm very encouraged that science is finally catching up with what women have always intuitively known. I recommend that, like Beverly, expectant mothers make tapes with words of love and encouragement to play for babies in their cribs and also in the womb. Or, you can play my *Embryos from the Heart* CD. A steady flow of positive vibrations and heartfelt words of encouragement will no doubt produce incalculable positive results.

Children can be very trying, and staying positive every minute of every day while taking care of them is almost an impossible task. But I urge you to try. I know it takes effort because I work very hard to keep my emotional state positive and pure. In fact, my heart is the generator behind the energy ray I use. I concentrate every waking moment to make sure that my heart is warm and tender, that I have only positive feelings for everyone I work with. It is why I get powerful results. If you achieve this, your vibrational rate will be very high and you will be a very positive person with a large energy field. Love is the strongest power, it's a builder, but negative energy creates explosion.

What to do with negativity that may arise in the course of family life? It's unconditional love that is expected as we evolve. Love and let live. Don't ever try to work out another's life program, even if you are in a deep relationship with them. If you cannot accept people as they are, do not become intensely involved with them. Do not for a moment think, "I can change that in them as our relationship develops." Acceptance, not expectation, is key. This is where so many unions go wrong.

Make an agreement with your partner, friends, and children who are old enough to understand that you won't dump negative emotions on one another. I believe that we have an inbuilt energy protection system, an instinct, to clear our energy fields of negative interference. People who dump on you leave you feeling exhausted and miserable because you have taken on their misery, whereas, they feel uplifted — not an equitable arrangement by any means. If you are aware that you are building up negative emotions, own every bit of your anger, frustration or hostility, and go to the woods or field or beach and turn it over to the Big Boss, as I call God. Scream and shake your fists and let it go. God can help you get rid of it. There's no judgment.

The Breath of Life (see page 120) is also useful for controlling your mind and temper. Take several deep breaths and recite affirmations to yourself that contradict the explosive situation at hand. "I'm strong and I can handle it," "My child is a sweet angel," or "My partner means well" might help you regain your composure, at least to the extent that you can calmly take charge of the situation. See your desired result as if it had already come about.

Don't forget that God is love. Your affirmations accompanied by positive emotions are seeds of perfect prayer. Divine energy responds to visualisation coupled with emotion, so say one affirmation at a time. Keep it as simple as possible and you'll be happily surprised with the results.

When I was in the Philippines I visited a church where prayers were answered on a regular basis. The place was so popular, you had to make a reservation months in advance to join the weekly intercessory prayer procession. I was amazed to see hundreds of women moving toward the altar on their knees, fervently praying and saying the rosary. Because they'd been waiting for so long to pray inside the church, they'd had ample time to visualise the desired result. Today there are many books on the power of visualisation and intention, but the knowledge has been around forever — and has produced excellent results.

Be sure to tell your loved ones about using these simple techniques so they have harmless outlets for their negative energy as well.

As I see it today, the problem is that children have boundless energy but many play areas have been eliminated. Homes have smaller yards and apartments have none. Children need to run and play on grass and beaches. They need to be exercised to burn huge amounts of energy. If they cannot do so, their energy turns negative from stress and frustration. I suggest that mothers make sure their children run and even run with them. They will eat well, be healthy, and sleep like babies.

Being fully and calmly in charge of your own situation is a necessary first step in making big improvements for everyone in the world.

At this time, and since 1994, power and responsibility for elevating the human race has shifted to women. We are in the early stages of an exciting transformation of consciousness that will advance humanity by 2000 years very quickly. If we can become aware of the vast power of our hearts and use it wisely and lovingly, we can create a world of peace, joy, and love for everyone's children to enjoy.

It all depends upon the power of love.

Chapter Eight

Frequency Wars

Finding a way to live comfortably in the UK had demanded constant effort on my part. The transition from my peaceful home in the woods to vibrant busy London kept me on my toes, energetically speaking. I was forever cleaning up the negative energy embedded in the walls of public places and clearing the lower frequencies of those around me before they dragged me down. Attending performances at London's renowned theatres and visiting historic attractions were challenging for me.

London has been the scene of devastating events dating back before Roman times. Vibrations from appalling scenes of public hangings, beheadings, stonings, and attacks by various groups throughout history have left negative frequencies implanted in the very walls of old buildings. Frequencies never die, so I could feel these frightening occurrences whenever I was near enough.

Negativity from World War II bombings by the Nazis still reverberates through large swaths of the city. Shock waves from more recent terror attacks by Irish extremists and large-scale attacks by Islamist fanatics still linger. Illegal immigration of unsavoury persons adds to the underlying gloom and fear that everyone feels at some level, though they try not to think about it. Almost half a million Londoners have moved away in recent years and immigrants are replacing them. Of course, most of the immigrants come looking for economic opportunity for themselves and their families, but a destructive element is moving in as well. When negativity builds beyond the point at which it can be contained, it must explode. An "about to explode" feeling pervades not just London but Paris and other major European cities.

I learned a good lesson about space and crowd cleansing when I was invited to Phantom of the Opera. I was particularly excited with the invitation, as it would be my first stage show in London. Every seat was taken in the huge theatre that seated hundreds of people. The performance was enthralling but by lunchtime the next day, I was so exhausted I had to cancel sessions with three clients and go to bed. The reason for my fatigue was obvious. While watching Phantom, I had exerted a great deal of energy working on the entire audience and cleaning the enormous theatre. In the effort to keep my personal environment clean and clear, I'd exhausted my reserves.

No one in London or other large metropolitan area can get away from the onslaught of manmade electromagnetic fields (EMF). Our bodies' own electrical fields interact with the electromagnetic fields of everything around us. Like every large city in the world, London is crisscrossed with high-voltage electrical power lines that keep lights, office equipment and home appliances running for millions of residents. Some people feel unpleasant "vibes" when walking under power lines but few are aware of the damage being done to their personal energy fields that may well lead to disease.

Far worse than the extremely low frequency (ELF) energy from power lines are wireless networks that run mobile phones and also wireless digital cameras and other handheld devices that every Londoner seems to carry.

Thankfully, the National Radiological Protection Board (NRPB) in England has been forced to admit that "electromagnetic hypersensitivity" (EHS) to electromagnetic frequencies can bring about fatigue, severe headaches and skin problems because of exposure to electromagnetic fields. One high-profile case was splashed all over the newspapers recently, bringing public attention to the problem. A successful businessman named Brian Stein, 55 year old CEO of a billion dollar UK company, has for several years been unable to cope with exposure to electromagnetic fields. His hypersensitivity first surfaced as severe pains in his ear when he began using mobile phones. He cannot ride in modern automobiles having electronic instrumentation or on electric trains, buses or long distance airplanes. He no longer watches television or listens to music on any device plugged into the wall.

The Swedes have recognised EHS as a physical impairment for years. They calculate that 3.1 percent of the population, 200,000 people, suffer from the condition. One Swedish experiment shows that there is an increase in mast cells near the surface of the skin when exposed to electromagnetic frequencies, a similar reaction to that when exposed to radioactive materials.

In spite of living in the midst of a sort of frequency war zone, my healing work progressed. My success was undoubtedly due to the constant work I did to keep my vibrations at a very high level. I wondered whether I might be able to transfer my vibrations to a CD for a wider circle of people to experience. The idea excited me and worried me at the same time. A CD could benefit millions of people, far more than I could possibly consult with one by one. But I couldn't be sure that my vibration would make its way through a maze of electronic equipment and onto the disc without getting contaminated. My phone sessions with clients worked beautifully, as telephone landlines are no problem. How would a CD work?

Rather than focusing on the why nots — and there were many — I sat down and wrote a script, found perfect background music, and signed up with a top-notch sound studio. I decided that my CD would be called *Dimensional Healing*.

When I decided to record my CD, *Dimensional Healing*,

I found being in the studio surrounded by electronic instruments was very complicated for me, as I could feel their different vibrations and had to keep warding them off. When I sat in the booth during the first recording session, put on earphones, and began speaking into the microphones, the overwhelming electric power kept on breaking my concentration.

I have trained myself to hold an unwavering focus, to attune to the highest vibrational level where my most powerful healing work is accomplished. I had to put forth an immense effort to overcome the competing vibrations in the studio and after each session, I worked hard for several days to boost my energy back to my usual vibrational level. Nevertheless, I was committed to making the effort to honour my deep intuitive knowledge that this CD was important. "I must be strong enough," I kept telling myself.

I have always had a rather unusual relationship with manmade power. Even during my teenage years in Australia, if I approached a flickering street lamp while on my evening walks, it would break down completely. This phenomenon continued in the USA. The power company box blew out on the house I was renting in Seattle when I got too close; and one time all the lights went out in front of a huge drugstore as I approached — I was at least a hundred feet from the entrance. In a bank in Seattle where I opened an account, the computer system crashed when

I walked in, much to the chagrin of the manager, who apologised profusely.

These occurrences were too regular to be coincidental. What was going on? I wanted to mend things in this lifetime, not destroy them. Thank goodness I was able to figure it out, even though it took many years. Now when my powerful positive energy comes into contact with an electrical device that has some sort of flaw, the weakness surfaces and my energy might go to work to mend it. In other words, I may find myself fixing electrical wiring, gadgets, and appliances the way I would clean a person's energy field and sometimes I don't even realise I'm doing it.

During the course of recording in the studio, an idea took shape and grew stronger with every session: My heartbeat belongs on the disc. My work is heart-centred and I want the vibration of love to come through. My heartbeat contains the vibration I work with and it was important to me to give it to the world. Also, because I exercise vigorously and keep my body in top-notch athletic condition, my heartbeat is strong and regular, providing a rhythmic pattern for listeners' hearts to follow. Scientists observed decades ago that hearts in close proximity tend to beat together, with the stronger one setting the pace.

I knew little of the technology involved, but the sound studio technician tried to reassure me. "Don't worry," he said, "I can put a drumbeat in that sounds like a heartbeat."

That wouldn't do at all. It had to be the beat of my heart. We were at an impasse. If the studio engineers couldn't figure out how to accomplish what I asked, the CD would just have to sit on the back burner until a solution was found. After weeks of doing my visualising prayer, it occurred to me to ask a nearby hospital for help. I had heard distinct heartbeats on medical documentaries on television. They had to have had the right equipment to get those sounds on tape.

I called Queen Charlotte Hospital, a maternity hospital, and ask to have a fetal monitor placed on my chest. Though my request was unusual, the staff didn't hesitate to book an appointment for me. I purchased a good recorder and set off.

The nurses could not have been lovelier. They lubricated my chest and ran the monitor over it as I lay on a bed. I turned on my recorder and lay still. "Gosh this is easy," I thought, remembering the last time I had been in a hospital decades earlier. "I don't even have to bear down this time, and it's painless."

We played it back before I left, and the results were perfect. The studio easily removed the sound of rushing blood and put the pure beat of my heart on the CD, accompanying my voice and the glorious music I'd found. Now I could give my heartbeat to the world.

Dr Jennifer Hunter, a physician in Australia, tested the CD with her patients and reported that many achieved "outstanding results" when using *Dimensional Healing*. Her patients "reported deep relaxation and often noted an improvement of symptoms." She also discovered that there is definitely a technology saturation point connected with my vibration. The purity of the vibration is ruined if the disc is played on a computer or downloaded from a computer to copy to a disc. If listeners are to get the full benefit, the CD must be played on a small CD player that is not attached to any other equipment.

I had my heartbeat put on my web site so people could hear a sample. As more people clicked on my site, I began to feel exhausted. It took months for me to realise that thousands of people were tapping into my heartbeat, and I was feeling it as though they were in session with me personally. When I'm working, I connect energetically to the client, almost like plugging an electric cord into a socket. If the healing is a heavy case, you can imagine the load I have to carry. But I've been prepared along the way to cope with weighty problems and though I may tire, I never feel anyone's needs as a burden. Rather, I'm excited and honoured to bring this work to the world, as I truly know that it's humanity's future healing method.

When *Dimensional Healing* at last came out, I was delighted with the number of emails I received telling me of its healing strength and meditation value. I was amazed at the number of people who mentioned that they listened to it over and over to be able to get through the program without falling asleep.

Healing of difficult problems occurred when the CD was left on continuous play next to their beds all night with the volume turned down. The healing vibration worked on their energy fields all night as they slept. Some people reported remarkable results when they left it on day and night to clear their physical space of negative frequencies. I'm honoured to have it available from the Nutri-Centre in London.

My next plan was to find an animator who could help me produce a film about the human energy field. Peter and his assistant had no idea of the existence of the field and found it difficult to visualise. A negative, unhealthy field was fairly easy for them, as it looks like television snow but the look of a healthy field was beyond their field of reference. Nevertheless they were to experience its effects in a surprising way.

I was exceptionally busy writing the script and didn't take much time to speak with them on a personal level. I was surprised when three weeks after Peter delivered the finished product, he called to thank me.

"I had a sick liver and was facing the possibility of a transplant. But new tests show that it's in perfect health. I want to thank you as I know my involvement with you and your work made the difference for me."

I was surprised and delighted of course. This healing happened on my unconscious level. Usually if I'm connected with someone person to person, I know of any illness they may have. In this instance, my concentration had been completely directed to getting my ideas across at our three meetings.

Another healing occurred with John, an animation producer. As we worked together, large, painful gallstones began to surface and become healed. It was fascinating to watch the progression of his animation. When the script got to the part where the gallbladder area is discussed, he illustrated with colours that were dark and dreary instead of the magnificent soft colours he used on the rest of the body. He was entirely unaware of why he had done so.

• • • •

It never ceases to amaze me that people have little understanding of energetic power, positive or negative. As I stated in *Conversations with the Body*, manmade energy is running counterclockwise, therefore, it's going against Earth's natural energy. By now, with our planet in such trouble, you'd think people would realise that we cannot continue to go against nature. But denial prevails.

Another common belief is that frequencies don't travel, that somehow they can be contained in the miles of electric wire that surround our homes, the places where we retreat to relax and re-energise. When you look at the modern Western home now, it probably contains three television sets, several computers, photocopiers, a fax machine, florescent lights which emit the strongest EMF, microwave ovens, vibrating electric lounge chairs, digital boxes to receive cable TV channels, video and DVD players, air-conditioners, and all-electric kitchens with every appliance plugged into the wall. An electronic security field probably surrounds all this. Even the dog wears a collar that buzzes with the signal from its very own electronic fence, discouraging it from crossing that invisible line — and doing God only knows what to its health. The garage has electronic doors and the car is computerised with many electronic extras such as security devices, television sets, DVD players, and even an electronic device to prevent rust.

Those who don't drive face their own share of problems on public transportation. According to a 2006 study by the World Health Organisation, you may be exposed to magnetic and electric fields in the passenger cars of long-distance trains and trams, with the greatest amount of power at floor level where motors and traction equipment are normally located. Some transportation systems powered by electricity expose riders to static magnetic fields, which are generated whenever electricity is used in the form of direct current (DC). In his excellent 1985 book, *The Body Electric*, physician Robert O. Becker tells us that "The starting and stopping of an electric train turns the power rail into a giant antenna that radiates ELF waves for over 100 miles."

Magnetic Resonance Imaging scanners, the popular

diagnostic tool known as MRI, also run on direct current and expose patients and hospital workers to very strong static magnetic fields. The WHO Study on Environmental Health Criteria published in 2006 states that direct current can generate electrical fields and currents around the heart and major blood vessels and slightly impede the flow of blood. They may also change "the orientation or position of biological molecules and cellular components" and interfere with certain types of chemical reactions that take place in the body.

Most people can't even get a good night's sleep anymore. They don't realise that their bedroom TVs and even their bedside lamps, radios, and clocks are bombarding them with unhealthy frequencies. Appliances are not really off when turned off by the switch; you have to pull the plug out fourteen inches from the socket to get the electrical frequencies to cease.

Though it's hard to generalise about the degree of danger a specific piece of electronic equipment presents, the cumulative effect is enormous.

Add the discordant frequencies of negative events that have taken place in certain locations and the overarching feeling of uncertainty that pervades the population on a daily basis and you can see how difficult it is for most people to keep their personal vibrations clear, their health sound, and their spirits high.

I haven't even begun to discuss the most dangerous

vibrations we're regularly exposed to. There's no question in my mind that mobile phone frequencies, vibrating at far higher rates than electrical appliances, are the most hazardous to health. They literally feed any weakness your body might have.

Mobile phone users surrounded me wherever I went in London. Whether they were sending or receiving calls, I saw small fusions form in people's fields, tangles of frequencies that are very hard to disentangle. It happens even when phones are turned off. I worked out a way to disentangle them fairly quickly, after which I needed to clean the circuits and put them back into their proper place in the field to make the pattern of the circuits strong again. You can imagine how busy I was in London every time I went out, as almost everyone in the city carries at least one mobile phone.

In Australia, a country of 19 million, 19 million mobile phones are registered; in England, there are millions more. The city of Shanghai, with its population of 18 million, has 16.3 million mobile phone subscribers. At this time, there are more than two billion in use worldwide — and the number rises daily.

Though a mobile phone might have a very low power output, it's not the power that's the problem. It's the frequencies. The higher the frequency of electromagnetic emissions, the greater the risk. Waves of electromagnetic energy vary in size, from very long radio waves the size of buildings (Low Frequency) to very short gamma rays smaller than atoms' nuclei (High Frequency). X-rays are the highest frequencies that most people are likely to come in contact with but fortunately exposure time is very short.

High frequencies are particularly dangerous for children. A recent study by the Spanish Neuro-Diagnostic Research Institute in Marbella revealed that high frequency electromagnetic waves emitted by mobile phones penetrated deeper into the brains of children than adults, with the deepest penetration occurring in the youngest subjects. Because children's skulls are thinner, a brief two-minute mobile phone call can interrupt the natural electrical activity of a child's brain for up to an hour afterwards. Physicians connected to the study worried that the resulting disruption to normal brain cell activity could cause children to lose their ability to concentrate, remember, and learn. Other radical changes might occur to mood and behaviour.

In Sweden, researchers at Lund University Hospital corroborated the findings of the Spanish study. Neurosurgeon Leif Salford and colleagues showed for the first time an unambiguous link between radiation emitted by GSM mobile phones and brain damage. Global System for Mobile Communications (GSM) is the most popular standard for mobile phones in the world with GSM service used by over 2 billion people across more than 212 countries.

The Swedish study also found that exposure to radiation emitted by mobile phones and neighbourhood relay towers can destroy cells in parts of the brain. "We can see reduced brain reserve capacity," Salford said. "...mobile phone radiation can allow harmful proteins and toxins to pass through the blood-brain barrier," thus posing a danger from certain medications that should not enter the brain. If certain proteins found in the blood can get to the brain, they may cause autoimmune diseases such as Fibromyalgia and Multiple Sclerosis.

The far-reaching consequences of mobile phone use are just beginning to be understood. Researchers and physicians in many parts of the world are concerned that prolonged exposure to radiation emitted by mobile phones and towers can bring on earlier Alzheimer's in people with a predilection for that dreadful disease. Other diseases are mentioned as well, like Parkinson's and cancer, brain cancer in particular.

In answer to public concern about the safety of mobile phones, manufacturers brought out earpieces to increase the distance between the phone and the subscriber's head. Problem was, they didn't work and in fact actually raised phone radiation risk. A *London Telegraph* article reported, "Using a model head filled with gel, researchers measured exposure levels behind the ear. In some tests, the ear piece increased exposure by up to 3-5 times."

A 2006 study conducted by prestigious Cleveland

Clinic in Ohio found that "men who used a mobile phone for more than four hours a day had a 25 percent lower sperm count than men who never used a mobile." Sperm quality was a problem as well, with swimming ability of sperm down by a third and a 50 percent drop in properly formed sperm.

I know of no study measuring women's fertility in relation to mobile phone use, but I can tell you that in my work with women trying to get pregnant, the adverse effects of mobile phone use are clear. I always make them promise to stay away from them and use landlines only during the course of their pregnancies. Women are especially sensitive to unnatural negative frequencies because of our higher vibrational level needed for reproduction.

The cover story on mobile phones in the October 9, 2000 edition of *Time* magazine ended with a warning from Lawrence Challis, vice chairman of the British group conducting extensive studies, "If there is a choice, use a landline phone."

In spite of mounting evidence, mobile phone companies continue to deny that they are causing multiple sclerosis, brain tumours, and permanent damage to the nervous system in children. You cannot avoid mobile phones now, as virtually every person travelling on public transport has one. Also, when your friends call you from their mobile phones, you are exposed to the frequencies. I won't speak to anyone who calls on a mobile and recommend that you tell your friends and family that you won't either. The frequencies are never truly off.

You can imagine the power of the wireless network, when London police were able to pull a switch to disconnect every person's phone during the terrorist attack in 2005. Terrorists love mobile phones and use them not only to communicate but also to detonate explosive devices. In my view, it's an example of negativity attracting negativity.

Even landline phones are not as clear as they once were, no matter where in the world you are calling. I cannot help wondering whether the problem is caused by increasing use of sophisticated radar mazes in the skies by various countries to detect incoming missiles. Not every country has an early warning system, but frequencies travel so we are all affected.

I do notice that my clients' energy fields are taking at least twice as long now to appear in my visualisation. As I mentioned earlier, my positive energy has to be at least three times as strong as the negativity I'm fighting.

• • • •

When I find fusions in a person's energy field caused by mobile phones, I know I am going to find inflammation flooding the immune molecule in the head, caused by sluggishness of head fluid flow during calls. I have a video produced by a company in Australia showing how the blood thickens during calls. Their research was done with the aid of medical doctors and scientists.

This molecule, representing the immune system, needs to be cleansed. Prolonged buildup from phone usage destroys the immune system. When flow is restored to the fluids and drainage resumes, my client may experience a brief period of discomfort such as headaches, neck problems, hearing problems, stinging eyes or blurry eyesight, and feelings of pressure in the head.

Lauri's story comes to mind, as radiation and poisoning related to her major illness. Initially, when I scanned her body, I detected a leak in her heart and used my ray to mend it. When she called the next week, she reported that her heart was calmer. Other symptoms pointed to chemical poisoning in her lungs affecting the heart and causing a tight chest. When I told her my findings, she replied that they explained mystery symptoms that her physician hadn't spotted "with all his machines."

I knew intuitively that she'd been in some difficulty for more than twenty years. She thought for a moment and recalled that she came down with glandular fever while redecorating her home many years previously. This explained the serious build up of poisons in her system — materials the builders had used on her home had been loaded with toxins. She also had a nasty virus in her liver along with parasites in her gut.

In addition to our healing sessions, I advised her to get a worming pill from her physician, take two tablespoonfuls of castor oil, get milk thistle to cleanse her liver, and take four baths a week with Epsom salts and vinegar to help her system detoxify. She faithfully followed my instructions and also did the Breath of Life five times a day and listened to her *Dimensional Healing* CD daily as well. Her health improved but she wasn't getting well as quickly as I'd expected. It occurred to me that her home might hold the answers.

Lauri lived in a lovely village, but I was certain it was contributing to her health problems. Sure enough, there were thirty huge pylons surrounding the house, airport radar and a farmer dusting poison around an adjacent field. Unbeknownst to me, she had actually paid an investigator two years previously to check out the area and after he'd taken readings and measurement with scientific instruments, he'd told her exactly what I told her. She'd have to move if she wanted to be healthy.

When Lauri finally moved to an area with fewer manmade frequencies to contend with, her health improved rapidly. She wrote to me saying that she'd been to the doctor and had received the all clear. Her blood pressure was normal, her blood work was perfect, her ulcer was healed, her sugar imbalance cured, the chemical poisoning was out of her system completely and her virus was gone.

• • • •

My heart goes out to the many people unwittingly

suffering from chronic environmental illnesses, most of which are undiagnosed. They go from doctor to doctor depleting their finances, looking for answers, and trying to restore their health. Few physicians have a clue that huge electrical junction boxes or mobile phone masts near their homes might cause their mystery maladies. Perhaps it's something as simple as chemical poisons from nearby farmers who spray crops.

I've seen people lose everything seeking an accurate diagnosis and effective treatment in their quest for health. Some even lose their homes, have no money left to move to healthier locales and no energy left to bring about a change. Because they cannot escape the radiation and poisons in their environments, they cannot become well.

If you fall into this category, seek outside support, help from friends or family. You have to find the courage and strength to save yourself.

● ● ● ●

On my annual trip home to Australia for Christmas, I was booked on a brand new plane that cut hours off the flight. I hadn't realised that this "wonderful" new design had a household size TV set on the back of the seat in front of me, just an arm's length away. Of course, the wiring was running through my backrest for the person behind. Every seat on the plane had a TV set embedded in it. I suppose I should have been grateful that use of mobile phones was banned on the plane. Since the time of this flight, Qantas and Emirates Air have begun to allow them for certain uses — and I have no doubt that other airlines will follow suit.

When I first arrived in Sydney I was fine. Then I started to go downhill as my field became absolutely drained, which took three days. I then became so ill my family thought I was leaving the planet. It took six weeks to recover. I have never felt as though I had no energy, I mean absolutely none, even during all my healing years after my car accident. Later I learned of other people with the same symptoms who literally died after a long flight. And recently I heard that a long flight can produce the same amount of stress in the body as playing four games of hockey.

When I was well enough to travel again, I returned on an older plane and had no problem. Coincidentally, the magazine tucked into the back of the seat in front of me bore the headline: "Cosmic Radiation, Do You Know The Risks?"

Actually, I worked with an airline pilot who knew the risks all too well. I was amazed when Dave called me from the Middle East. He'd found my book in a little shop in Dubai and wanted to tell me about his health problems. An international airline captain, he had had an exciting life but had recently been diagnosed with malignant skin cancer that caused him to lose his flying licence. He described feeling "emotionally empty, tired, being without energy."

Dave discovered research studies on the Internet by

doctors investigating the health problems of men in his line of work. A University of Iceland study showed "a high occurrence of malignant melanoma among commercial airline pilots." Several possible contributing causes were cited: Pilots were subjected to cardiovascular stress from irregular hours and crossing of time zones, ongoing exposure to high-output energy fields of radar, radios and generators, natural background radiation especially above 30,000 feet, low air pressure, hours of noise and UV light exposure among other stresses.

When we first talked, I could hear the exhaustion in Dave's voice. Without hesitation I sent one of my MP3 players to boost his energy. Even before we had private sessions, he reported "after listening to this program on a regular basis I could actually feel changes taking place. I became less tired, more relaxed, less negative in my expressions and opinions and better able to emotionally handle my disease." I had to smile about his still being surprised with himself for contacting me even after his skin started to clear up.

It's very interesting how positive and negative energies relate to weight. Positive energy is white in colour and weightless. Enlightened people are optimistic, positive and have an approach to life that is light both in colour and weight. On the other hand, negative energy is heavy from all the negative frequencies we have given birth to not only from dark, pessimistic thoughts and feelings but also from the technological products we fill our lives with.

Poor management of the Earth's resources may weigh upon us as well. At some level, though we may be careful recyclers and promoters of environmental causes, we may feel guilt and regret for the damage humankind has done. We have a chance to lift vibrations by insisting on clean energy. I love the white windmills I've seen dotting the landscape of many countries during my travels and wind turbines that produce power. Not only is their colour correct but they are also in harmony with earth energy. Denmark is leading the way toward switching to windmill power with now almost a quarter of their energy needs are provided by wind turbine energy — and plans in the works for gradually phasing out fossil fuels. Wherever you live, you can take an active part in calling your government's attention to the possibilities in your country.

Though we have a long way to go, we can look forward to a time when our energy is produced in harmony with the natural heartbeat of Earth. Stress would be eliminated in every living thing and nature would be happy again, especially if we stop cutting down so many trees. As we have seen in the climate changes and powerful natural disasters in recent years, Mother Nature is in distress, to say the least. You cannot go against the grain of nature without consequence. When nature reacts, it's with tremendous power, negative in expression. We're helpless against the might of wind and water. I can't understand why the 21st

Centurion cannot get to the bottom line, to fix the problem that's creating so much destruction and suffering.

We are in the midst of a war of frequencies that few people acknowledge, and the negative is winning. My major concern about the buildup of negative frequencies is that the weight of them could add to the tilt the planet already has and cause it to flip. Ancient predictions of a devastated dying planet could become a reality.

Is it too late? Beyond our control or influence? Perhaps. But we must give it our all. Remember, God, the universal Divine wisdom, responds to prayers said from the heart with the full force of your emotions invested in them.

The Ultimate Spa Experience

Very soon, I'll see the work I'm doing incorporated into spas and health clubs, which are already pampering the outside of the body. This vibrational healing will pamper the inside too, making this beautiful method the total package. You'll come away from a trip to the spa truly healthier in every way. In a sense, these will be our future hospitals, though conventional hospitals will still exist for surgery and other procedures.

• • • •

Chapter Nine

Electronic Bugs

I shall never forget my first sighting of a worm in a person's liver. I was shocked. I thought I must be mistaken. Was I losing it? Later that day, a friend's husband came to the rescue of my confidence.

"You will never believe what I saw in a liver this morning," I said, "worms! I think my imagination is working overtime."

Roger had recently retired and sold his butcher shop. "Your imagination is not the problem, Robyn," he said, "I saw them many times in animal livers."

Over the last three years I've become increasingly aware that parasites are evolving faster than before, becoming more prevalent and harder to eradicate. Intestinal worms are invading great numbers of people. A study reported in The American Journal of Tropical Medicine and Hygiene revealed that 32 percent of a "nationally representative sample of 2,896 people" tested positive for infection. Clearly, you no longer need to leave home to catch them, but it's hard to find a doctor who'll test for them unless you've just stepped out of a steaming jungle.

Few Western physicians studied parasitology, as until recent years, infestations were rare. But now outbreaks have been reported in 48 of the 50 US states. Once considered a third-world problem, today, more than 125 different species of parasites live in North American food supplies, water, air, and the soil.

Parasites make their way around the globe with travellers who've been on adventure vacations to exotic locales and businessmen and women returning from global business trips. In any international airport you might brush up against persons carrying not only their luggage but also infectious parasites and disease causing organisms. And planes take on catering deliveries from other countries, including raw salad ingredients that may or may not have been properly washed. Probably the greatest source of parasites is from produce grown in developing countries and then imported into the markets of non parasite areas.

Viruses and bacteria have also found ways to become more invasive than ever. Over-use of antibiotics has created resistant strains of bacteria with sometimes deadly and potentially catastrophic results. The new "superbug," methicillin-resistant staphylococcus aureus (MRSA) is now roaming the streets, having found its way off hospital walls. It is resistant to all penicillin antibiotics.

Tapeworms and roundworms are breeding faster and laying twice as many eggs. Exotic worms are also hitchhiking in great numbers from developing countries' seafood farms to take up residence in the human populations of the UK, the USA, Canada and every other country in the world that imports food. Speedy airline delivery quickly puts them on your table.

Eggs of worms found in seafood, especially in shrimp, have a longer life than the parent who laid them. You don't even have to eat the fish to become ill, as those who work growing, shipping, and handling these infested products are also at risk. For this reason, I never eat raw fish myself, like sushi, and I don't think you should either.

The family dog and cat and other animals may also be infected. I know one brand of premium cat food that features whole shrimp in a fancy pâté. I'd want to know where those pretty little shrimp came from before feeding it to my pet.

A handful of scientists have put forth the theory that the newfound power of these invaders comes from adapting their biological frequencies to those emitted by computers and especially the mobile phone. This is not yet a widely accepted theory but my experience in eradicating parasitic invaders from my clients has shown me that it's true. Parasitic invaders have frequencies that are becoming virtually electronic and are slipstreaming on the waves electronic equipment emits. This is probably the reason that antibiotics and other medical treatments don't reliably work against them.

Once they gain entry to the body, parasites make their way to the digestive tract with many heading directly into the liver. Once parasites destroy the liver, they hold full power to destroy human life. I advise my clients to get a prescription for worm medicine — the only time I advise using a strong chemical in the human body.

The only way to destroy them would be to use an electronic zapping device yet to be developed. Biophysicist Hilda Clark was aware of this when she invented a "zapper" for worms — and of course was threatened by the US government for doing so. I do hope she has strengthened her electronic instruments to keep up with the increasing power of parasites.

The majority of sick people now contacting me have either a worm or virus in their bodies. Their medical practitioners have not been able to give them accurate diagnoses because they don't think to look for parasites and even if they do, worms are very good at camouflaging themselves to blend with human and animal flesh. Tapeworms lie flat against flesh, hooking on with barbs. I pick them up only because my ray makes them move. Viruses can easily be missed as well. The hepatitis virus settles into the liver and makes itself at home in small labyrinths.

Recently, I discovered that the viruses I kill and eradicate can leave a small reproduction of themselves as a calling card. This has always been the case with worms, which deposit their eggs as they die, but I had not seen this with a virus previously. I was so surprised when it came up in my visualisation while working on a client, I phoned Dr John Walck for his input. After a moment of thought he answered, "Yes they could reinvent their cells."

For years I have been saying, "They can scrub hospital walls with soap and disinfectants all day and night. They will not get rid of these electrical bugs." In the past MRSA infections stayed in hospitals but a recent study of 2000 cases found that 30 percent developed outside health care settings. Now we see articles with headlines: "Warning! Dreaded Hospital Scourge Threatens Public."

Chilling warnings are issued by the US Center for Disease Control and Prevention (CDC) alerting the public to dreaded MRSA staph infections continually finding new ways to spread. The cleaning of floors and walls needs to be done by electric vibrational machine, more powerful than soap and water. Previously, patients became infected when they had an open wound or their skin was broken in some way. Now bacteria have evolved so a patient can become infected without any break in the skin.

MRSA have also found ways to acquire a gene that makes them even more invasive. A person can now become infected with the superbug without setting foot in a hospital, as cases are originating in gymnasiums, prisons, nursing homes, schools, military bases, and tattoo parlors. MRSA can even be sexually transmitted.

In the Netherlands, pig farms have become a source of infection, with MRSA bacteria carried from pigs to humans. Worldwide, an estimated 53 million people carry MRSA. Skin contact is the usual point of infection, however MRSA has recently been observed in a form that can spread through the air.

Healthy people infected with MRSA may carry it around for years without developing symptoms. Infections may initially look like a spider or insect bites. Boils and abscesses can develop. In the worst case, these can turn into necrotising fasciitis, the dreaded flesh-eating disease that maims and often kills. A recent tragic case in the Seattle area involved a darling little six-year-old boy with the most engaging smile, who bumped his lip while playing ball at school. Within a few days, the scrape turned into a staph infection that quickly became a full-fledged case of necrotising fasciitis. Only by cutting away much of the tissue of his face and head did physicians manage to save his life. No family should have to go through such a nightmare.

You have to be vigilant and take precautions. The CDC reports that hand washing would save lives of about 30,000 people in the US annually. Alcohol is an effective hand sanitiser, and I recommend always carrying little packets of alcohol-soaked towels available at the drugstore. Be sure to give a supply to your children. Wash your hands frequently when you touch things in public places. Also, tell them to use only their own towels and athletic equipment. Keep injuries clean. Seek treatment early, especially if a fever develops. Make sure health care providers wear gloves before they examine you, as their last patient may have been a MRSA carrier.

E.coli is another highly contagious bug that is running rampant in places we never dreamed of, such as ATM machines and on women's cosmetic purses and make-up containers. I find it hard to eat in restaurants, except for a few I believe are as clean as my home. One thing I'd like to see is the people who have cooking shows on TV wearing lightweight plastic gloves while demonstrating their recipes. They could influence countless viewers to follow good food-handling practices.

According to the British Journal of Biomedical Science, diarrhoeal illness continues to be a major public health burden worldwide. Once a rare occurrence, E.coli has emerged as a leading cause of food-borne illness in developed countries in recent years, with a number of large outbreaks reported. The CDC explains that E.coli infection often leads to bloody diarrhea, abdominal cramps, and occasionally to kidney failure.

Some meat may become contaminated during slaughter, and organisms can be accidentally mixed into meat. Undercooked ground beef has caused the greatest number of E.coli outbreaks. People have also become ill from E.coli found in sprouts, lettuce, spinach, salami, unpasteurised milk and juice. Drinking and bathing water can be a problem as well if it is contaminated by sewage. In some restaurants in places where health department rules are lax, bathrooms and kitchens share the same piping, thus creating a perfect avenue of contamination if there are any leaks or breaks in the pipes. Farm animals and those in petting zoos can carry E.coli right into your children's loving arms. The bacteria can contaminate the ground, railings, feed bins, and fur of the animals.

We now have to be cleaner than ever, but try not to let paranoia set in, as it can be damaging as well. Let common sense prevail.

A lovely young woman named Nicci became a client a year and a half after she returned from a visit to South America. She and her partner had gone for a holiday and she'd begun to feel ill four days after they arrived. When they returned, Nicci's condition continued to deteriorate over 18 months.

Every night she experienced chronic nausea and vomiting; every day her stomach felt terrible. Her complexion turned a jaundiced yellow colour. Only 5 feet 2 inches tall, she lost 75 pounds and dreaded looking in the mirror. She sought out two top surgeons in her city, had diagnostic tests including three endoscopies, but the doctors could not come up with a diagnosis. They suspected a liver problem but could not find a cause. Finally they threw up their hands and told Nicci it was all in her head, including the yellow skin! Nicci then turned to alternative and natural healers, to no avail.

A friend of hers found *Conversations with the Body* in a bookstore a few days before Nicci planned to commit suicide. She'd already organised her business and personal effects. When she called she sounded dubious about my method of healing but felt I was her last resort. We went ahead.

When I started scanning her body, I saw that her gallbladder was shriveled. Her knees showed weakness and her head had a nasty bump on it. But by far the worst problem in Nicci's body was her liver, which was in a terrible state. By the end of the third treatment I suspected that a stomach ulcer was also part of the problem.

During the fourth treatment while doing my usual scanning, I suddenly realised that the thing I'd tentatively identified as a stomach ulcer had come to the fore. It turned out to be a 6-inch long worm.

It was the first time I had encountered a worm of this size. I was actually horrified, as I thought I was looking at an infection collecting around an ulcer and was about to treat it in my usual way, using the ray as a hook to pull out infection. I didn't expect to see a worm. Obviously I had disturbed it. It's movement came as a shock.

I always try to maintain a professional attitude with my work, but I have to admit this was one occasion that I lost it. "My God, it's a worm!" I exclaimed. By now I was three inches down. "Measure," I thought, "six inches now." I went underneath and up the other side, not knowing exactly how to proceed. I did know I had to kill it. I did so by dissecting its head. "Watch for the elimination of this creature. You should see its departure."

Our session took place at 11:00 a.m. Six hours later, I thought I should check Nicci to see if it had left. It's very useful to be able to instantly go to the body part I have been working with to check its progress. To do that, I mentally recall the client's voice, even just one word. Then I can dive into the body part. This ability is particularly valuable when I'm draining inflammation and infections; they need to be kept moving, as build-up creates discomfort.

I have no idea and don't want to know what the client is doing at the time of my follow-up visits, as I have no intention of invading their privacy. I don't see the outside of the body, just the organs I'm working on. This time I was checking to see if this worm had left. It was still there, although, I could tell it was dead by its colour and the state of its tissue. Why wasn't it gone? When I proceeded to go to its end to use my hook, I noticed barbs attaching it to the wall of the intestine. I swear as a minister, I did not know the biological make up of these worms previously, so I didn't know what I was looking at. Barbs? Legs? Did she swallow a centipede? I was completely baffled.

I started the job of removal, digging them out of the flesh. This was exhausting, I could only remove one set at a time. I took fifteen-minute breaks to renew my concentration, as it was very difficult, demanding work.

The following week, Nicci reported having had diarrhea for two days. During that time she was amazed to pass the worm in three sections, which proved my measurements. A week later, I was able to kill the eggs and remedy other effects of this worm. I advised her to go to the pharmacy for worm medicine. She bought everything they had on the shelves — perhaps too enthusiastically, but Nicci tells me that she is now in perfect health.

I talked to physicians I knew about what kind of worm it might have been. My description led them to believe it was what is commonly known as a pork tapeworm.

•••

Davinda was a client in the UK I had worked with five years earlier. She called to ask for my help again.

"Robyn, I think you should have a look at me, my husband and I have been trying for a baby but I don't feel well, and my energy is very low."

My scan revealed the dreaded worm in her liver, the same worm I'm finding in so many livers now that come from Asian seafood farms. It's being labeled the "exotic worm."

"You're blessed not to have become pregnant, Davinda." It would only be worse if we'd found the worms after she'd become pregnant.

Like others who are infested with parasites, Davinda experienced bloating in the digestive system. I wanted her to get the parasites out of her system as soon as possible. There are herbal preparations that purportedly remove parasites gently and gradually, but I've found that most people don't follow a regular schedule with them and some even forget to continue taking them before the required dosage is taken.

On our first sessions, I eradicated as many parasites as possible in Davinda's intestines and her liver, which would need to be stronger in order to tolerate the powerful chemical in the worming medicine. When she was strong enough, she took the first dose. The liver purged infection and I kept cleaning for about three weeks. I also located and removed some eggs during this time. To ensure that all parasites were eradicated, I recommended a backup dose for the sake of complete cleanliness. Once the infection went, the liver strengthened and labyrinths began to heal.

At this stage, Davinda (and my other clients with the same condition) pick up very quickly. Their livers are regenerated and wellness is established.

I have not and will not divulge the name of the product I use because unless monitored, it can have a dangerous effect on a weakened liver. But you can ask your physicians to prescribe anti-parasitic medication for you. My work strengthens the liver so it can tolerate the dose.

So far, my approach to parasite eradication has had

complete success. Medication for even the common thread and pinworm is still hard to buy over the counter in the USA. Australia and South Africa in the western world led the way I believe, making medication available for forty or more years. An even stronger treatment can now also be purchased in Australia. The United Kingdom is also marketing over the counter worm treatment for easy availability.

A major problem now is that these bugs are developing in strength so quickly. They are attuned to the frequencies of mobile phones and computers and other electronic products, which are becoming stronger as well. Any medication or products needed to combat them continually have to be strengthened to have an effect.

• • • •

Cindy, whom I helped with her pregnancy in Chapter 7, "Embryos From The Heart," called again two years later to ask me to help her and her husband conceive another baby. I told her I didn't think she needed my help, that the new child would be conceived naturally because of our previous work.

Six months later, Cindy called with good news. She was pregnant. "I'm still nervous though, so I hope you will work with me."

While scanning during our first session, I could see exactly why she felt the need of my help again. It was purely instinctual on her part to ask for support, as her liver was riddled with exotic worms. Not pinworms or round worms, but the same variety I've seen repeatedly riding in on shrimp or prawns from seafood markets in Asia. I was not surprised to learn that Cindy loved shrimp and had been eating a lot of them.

This exotic worm is different. It sets up homemaking labyrinths in the liver for its purpose. They create huge amounts of infection filled with a nasty breed of bacteria. As fast as I attack them with my ray they breed up quickly again from hatching eggs deposited as they are dying. The instinct of the worm is to use its body as a host. Its main objective is to breed by getting the eggs out of its body. I have seen a beheaded worm still laying eggs in the intestines and livers.

Unsurprisingly, Cindy's heart was also in trouble. When these worms invade, many organs are weakened. The host's liver becomes too weak to cleanse the blood efficiently. Unclean blood affects the heart, which in turn weakens. The weakened liver cannot produce enough bile and digestive systems from stomach to bowel slow down. Digestive systems under attack produce gas, bloating and pain. Cindy was no exception. Like others carrying this worm, she had most of these symptoms. Left untreated, it could only get worse.

Some doctor might have suggested abortion and encouraged her to clean out and start again, but I knew her too well for that. It would have broken her heart. She was a loving mother who really wanted another baby. This baby.

I knew I could not give her the strong chemicals I recommended to others for these worms, as it would abort the embryo. What a dilemma. The pressure was on. Our only hope was for me to somehow find the power to get on top of the worms and eventually eradicate them. The main problem was to keep them from entering the placenta. The strain on me was tremendous.

In the end, Cindy gave birth to a healthy baby boy. It was hell for me, however. I scanned baby at four weeks of age, holding my breath that he was clear. I thanked God that he was, and Cindy was able to safely breastfeed her new child.

Progress on the Pacific Coast

"If you can enter the space between cells and molecules or the spaces among molecules, you will experience being in another dimension. At that time, you will find it also a boundless dimension."

Master li Hongzhi
Falun Zuan

Chapter Ten

Animals Also Evolve

When I was a child I started my healing journey by binding up paws of neighbourhood pets. Later I learned to communicate psychically with some of the horses I trained. Those who read my last book will know about Fred, the wonderful horse who helped my head injuries to heal. I'm not surprised to learn that horses are now being used for rehabilitation of addicts and also for the disabled, who gain confidence as they learn to ride. I've always loved animals, feel connected to them, and have great respect for their great hearts and intelligence.

You can imagine how touched I was by reports of lovely Capuchin monkeys being trained as companions and helpers for quadriplegics. Helping Hands, an organisation in Boston, trains the intelligent little monkeys to do everyday jobs like brushing hair or taking a bottle from the refrigerator, unscrewing the top, and handing it to the person. Besides performing many useful tasks, the good-natured primates provide loving companionship that helps dispel clouds of boredom and depression for their humans.

I cannot bear to think of all the primates who have lost their lives because people kill them for sport, for their meat or for fur. One type of Capuchin is facing extinction in Brazil because of loss of habitat as the rain forest is methodically chopped down and burned. The slaughter of chimpanzees and gorillas in Africa is horrific. Gorilla parts are sold still as trophies. The loggers who are destroying their habitat are eating chimpanzees. The intelligence of a chimp equals that of a six-year-old human child, which adds to the horror. Some wonderful humanitarians in Africa are saving babies who are left motherless, but it's not a perfect solution, as these unfortunate babies can never be returned to the wild.

Many efforts by well-meaning environmental scientists to tag wildlife with tracking devices are questionable. What are tranquilising drugs and electronic collars and chips doing to the animals? Knowing what I do about electrical frequencies, I rather doubt they get off without serious negative effects. It would seem that mankind would not be happy until they are all gone, except a few remaining in zoos.

Whales and dolphins have been beaching themselves in great numbers all over the world. For one reason, manmade electrical fields interfere with their natural sonar systems and confuse them until they don't know which signals to respond to. In 2004, there was a mass stranding of more than 150 melon-headed whales at Hanalei Bay on my favourite Hawaiian island, Kauai. At that time, a study by National Oceanic and Atmospheric Administration (NOAA) concluded the whales — which usually inhabit only deep water — may have heard sonar signals from Navy ships in the area and headed into the shallow water.

I was enormously pleased that in June 2006, President Bush designated the Northwestern Hawaiian Islands as a marine national monument where marine life could not be disturbed. My hopes were quickly dashed when, before the end of that month, the US Navy received a federal permit to conduct new sonar testing exercises there after NOAA said that "use of the sonar is not likely to jeopardise the continued existence of threatened and endangered species — including the Hawaiian monk seal — in the exercise areas." It was a bureaucratic nightmare of epic proportions with lives of hundreds of sea creatures in the balance until a private environmental organisation, Natural Resources Defense Council, filed a lawsuit. Their senior attorney Joel Reynolds said it was "absurd to designate an area a marine national monument one week, and then authorise the Navy to blast it with high-intensity sonar the next." By the time the environmentalists prevail — if they ever really do — it may be too late for marine mammals. Some environmental scientists predict the end of sea life by the year 2040. I cannot imagine a planet having no sea life left.

The very same bureaucrats who decided to allow sonar testing might take their families to swim with the dolphins on their next vacation, never stopping to ask themselves why they feel so much better afterwards. If they are ill, they may well experience rapid healing after their time with the dolphins, but they cannot understand it as simple cause and effect. Dolphins are loving creatures with very high-level vibrations. They want to pattern the human field vibrations after their own. They clear the energy fields of humans who swim with them automatically and lift them into their own vibrational zone. Living in their high-vibration zone is responsible for dolphins being such happy and joyous animals.

In Africa and Asia majestic elephants are in danger of extinction. At the rate of decline in elephant population it's estimated they will be extinct in only fifty years, as poachers and ivory hunters slaughter them for their tusks. Smaller than their African cousins, wild Asian elephants are even more persecuted through hunting and habitat loss with fewer than 50 thousand elephants remaining in the wilds of the Indian subcontinent and Southeast Asia, a fraction of their former population. Elephants are poisoned by plantation workers, shot by farmers, and killed for their meat and hide, as well as their tusks. According to the World Wide Fund for Nature, ivory poaching may be causing Asian elephants to lose the gene that allows them to develop tusks. About 40 to 50 percent of Asian elephants are normally tuskless, but in Sri Lanka, more than 90 percent of the population is not growing tusks.

"When you have ivory poaching, the gene that selects for whether an elephant has tusks or not will be removed from the population," said Paul Toyne, a species conservation officer of the WWF.

"In Uganda, African elephants are also evolving into tuskless animals. An article about these tuskless elephants in a September 1998 article in *The Daily Mail* states: "At one national park in Uganda, for example, there were 3,500 tuskless elephants in 1963. Thirty years later there were just 200. Today the population is 1,200 and growing rapidly.

The tuskless phenomenon has been chronicled by researchers at Queen Elizabeth National Park in Uganda. (www.mweyalodge.com/html/inthenews.html) A survey in 1980 recorded that only one percent of elephants were without tusks, as a result of a rare genetic mutation.

Now Dr Eve Abe, a Cambridge educated elephant specialist with the Government of Uganda, says that 15.5 percent of female elephants and 9.5 percent of the males in the park are tuskless.

Evidence is coming in that the tuskless elephant is occurring all over Africa, and particularly in southern Tanzania, where poaching levels are high."

• • • •

There is no doubt that dogs have evolved to incredible heights. We've all encountered seeing eye dogs in the street helping vision impaired people. Other dogs are trained to act as ears for the deaf and to fetch and carry things for those who cannot do those tasks for themselves. Their keen sense of smell makes them ideal for detecting explosives in war zones and drugs at airports. I was so impressed with the wonderful work that dogs can do that I joined the Guide Dog Association, a worthwhile charity in London, as I wanted to support their work.

Now, dogs are being taught to read. A veteran dog trainer Dr Bonnie Bergin, President of the Assistance Dog Institute in Santa Barbara, California, wrote a book *Teach Your Dog To Read*. She states that with her technique, most dogs that respond to verbal commands can learn to read three words in 15 minutes. With practice dogs can learn as many as twenty words.

She suggests that you print a word representing an action such as SIT in large dark letters on a piece of white paper. Hold the card behind your back while your dog is standing.

Pull the card out, hold it in front of you and say, "sit." Your dog should see the word before he hears the command. When the dog sits, say, "yes, good dog" and reward him. Repeat three or four times and most dogs will sit when they see the card. Repeat the process in new training sessions using a new word.

My first doggie client was Elliot, my friends' companion animal. Jane and Michael had tried to do everything right for him. He'd been on a raw food diet since he was three months old, and thrived on it until he was two and a half years old.

Suddenly he began having stomach problems with bouts of severe diarrhea for a few days. It would clear up and then return a week or two later. The family had moved to a different state, and his new vet did not believe in the raw diet. She blamed it for Elliot's diarrhea and sent him home. Jane cooked his food for a while, but he still had bouts of diarrhea.

Jane contacted a pet psychic who said that Elliot had something sharp and solid like a piece of bone lodged in his colon near his pelvis. This was causing an obstruction that left the area around it inflamed and infected. She suggested barium enemas and diagnostic tests and predicted he would need surgery to remove the obstruction.

That's where the situation stood when Michael and Jane picked me up for dinner one night to discuss another matter. Elliot was in the car, but wasn't sure yet that I was his new best friend.

When they told me about Elliot I felt certain that I could help him. I was sure I could get in and out before Elliot knew I was there. But the moment I went in, he felt me and jumped back. I found the piece of bone lodged in his colon, and moved it sufficiently to allow it to pass. After dinner, I took another look and felt confident that it was indeed moving along.

Soon the bone passed out of Elliot's system naturally and he was free from its effects. Jane and Michael later confirmed that Elliot remained well and did not have any more attacks.

Elliot was an easy case for me. Animals are totally unselfconscious, trusting, honest, and a joy to help.

Jane and Michael are model pet owners but many dogs suffer because owners treat them as persons, dress them in silly outfits, and carry them around like babies. Living an apartment lifestyle is unnatural. I know many are taken for walks, but they would exercise much more if they could be outside in a large space all day. Dogs need to be able to run constantly.

Much of the canned food they are fed is not the best thing for them. To underscore the fact, six million cans and pouches of cat and dog food contaminated with rat poison from China were recalled recently but not before a reported 500 pets were poisoned to death. Under the best conditions, though there's quite a difference in canned pet food from brand to brand and country to country, none is ideal. Dogs are carnivores who need fresh raw meat and bones to thrive (except chicken bones). Few dogs are lucky enough to have perfect lives with fresh meat and large yards. Obesity is a major problem with dogs, as it is with humans, and for exactly the same reasons — the wrong food and too much of it, and not enough exercise.

Veterinary care is very expensive. Usually the

veterinarian's approach is quite good, as it is still very connected to the natural healing ability of the animal's body. I'm not sure about other countries, but I've heard that in Australia, students have a harder time getting into veterinary colleges than they do into medical school. Vets do not immediately use chemicals to numb the animal's ability to heal, which is often what physicians do when patients come to them asking them to "give me something for this pain, Doc." In many ways, veterinarians have an easier job than physicians do as few of their patients carry emotional baggage and can heal faster. Animals just get on with it.

Vets have always known that, left untreated, worms will kill. But it's hard to convince physicians to test for worms and parasites. I can't believe that medical doctors and their patients are still in denial about this growing problem. Most Americans are aghast when I tell them they need worm treatment. "Humans don't have worms," they reply. Vets have a device that can detect worms almost instantaneously. With the trillions spent on medical research, one would think that a small amount could be directed toward devising a human version.

I often have seen people kissing their pets on the mouth and allowing them to lick their lips. If you're ever tempted to get all kissy with Fido or Fluffy, try to remember where their little pink tongues have been. I love and adore animals, but don't let us all get confused here.

But you don't have to kiss them to get parasites, as parasite eggs are deposited everywhere, on carpets, chairs, clothing, and even in your car. It's a wonder that worms don't invade more people. Both humans and pets get the same chemical agent as a remedy for worms, but because so many doctors are in denial about worms invading their patients, it's almost impossible to obtain a prescription.

Things are looking up, however, with newspapers and magazines increasingly writing about the growing invasion of worms and parasites in even the best cared-for human bodies.

I seem to attract small bitey creatures whenever I get serious about writing. When I wrote *Conversations with the Body* in Hawaii, a centipede caused a frightening lesion on my foot that I had to work hard to get rid of. This time in Mexico, during my first day of writing, a persistent wasp kept buzzing over my shoulder. "Go away!" I said. It went. "Good, that worked," I thought, and forgot all about it.

A minute later, I felt a movement on top of my leg under my sarong. A powerful sting quickly answered my hasty brushing movement. Not very friendly, my wasp. I hadn't intended to hurt it and in fact it flew away. I know wasp bites can be ferociously toxic, but I had no particular problem with this one.

Soon after I got home, a client named Jim called from North Queensland hoping I could help him eradicate the poison in his body from not one, but two attacks from swarms of paper wasps while he was working in his garden. These insects caused him tremendous itching. It would take a long time for the injected poison to leave his body.

Jim had found my book in a Sydney bookstore and after reading it, called me for help. He was a vigorous middle-aged man who ate well, exercised regularly, took nutritional supplements, and in recent years lived a healthy lifestyle. In earlier years, however, he'd worked as a printer and had taken in a great many toxins that had built up in his system. Now retired, he occasionally helped his son at the print shop.

Jim had been exposed to the flu virus, but felt it would not take hold. However, within an hour of going to work in the print shop, his system "capitulated" and he was taken ill. He threw it off quickly, but a week later he had a rash all over his chest that spread over his entire torso, then down the limbs. The rash became "progressively worse until the itching was quite unbearable."

Jim's naturopath was unable to give him any relief, so he was forced to seek help from the medical profession. The doctor gave him cortisone cream, which he was trying desperately to avoid. The cream worked but the moment he stopped using it, his skin condition was back with a vengeance, actually worse than before. Jim had to move into the spare bedroom so his wife could sleep, as he was getting up several times a night to take long showers to give himself some respite.

At this point, Jim called me and we started to work. Having read *Conversations*, he knew what to expect and was very cooperative. He told me,

"If I had any doubts at all they were soon dispelled when you started assessing my field and checking me out. Things that only I knew about, such as a shoulder that can slip out (dislocate) as I roll over in my sleep. A scar behind my right ear, the result of a mastoid operation when I was 4 years old. A bad knee. My lower spine and an upper neck vertebrae that had recently been revealed as fusing in a scan I had been given were all identified as places she would have to work on."

I also found a lot of fluid in Jim's head that needed draining. It had been there since he'd been hit in the head with a golf ball twenty years previously.

When I scanned Jim's organs, I found his digestive and cardiovascular systems in fairly good working order. His lymphatic system, sinus system and endocrine systems were in trouble and his pituitary gland was quite unhappy. Alarming but not overwhelming his lungs and liver however were in dire straits.

I found a virus in his liver that was so entrenched it must have been there for ten or twelve years. It looked like Hepatitis. When I mentioned this to Jim he recalled having a course of inoculations when he purchased a hotel a dozen years earlier and was considered to be at risk from whatever might be floating around contaminating the old building. Eradicating the virus from his liver would take a great deal of work.

His lungs were in serious trouble, so severe that on my second visit, I actually blurted out that they were so full of toxins, he was lucky to be alive. He told me then that he had been a farmer as a young man, and then returned to that occupation for a while more recently. As a young farmer he hadn't taken proper precautions when using and handling poisons and was often soaked in them as he sprayed sheep for fly strike, dipped cattle for ticks, and sprayed crops.

Jim's system was already severely compromised by poisons accumulated over the years so when the wasps attacked, his toxic load hit critical mass. He couldn't tolerate even a small amount of additional poison, including drugs he might have been given that produced the slightest side effect. Thank goodness he hadn't taken more medication than the cortisone cream. As I pared away toxins from Jim's lungs and the rest of his system, I had to tell him his skin would become more irritated than ever until they were flushed out of his system. The skin is the largest organ in the body and does a major job of eliminating toxins.

Jim did his part like a trooper, taking castor oil to keep the toxins moving in the colon, bathing his feet in a bucket of warm water containing 50 drops of iodine to assist with toxin purging, and taking long soaks in the bathtub with Epsom salt and vinegar.

Jim found it almost impossible to buy tincture of iodine

in Australia. Once a standard in medicine chests all over the world, iodine seems to be disappearing. It's one of the once-common health products that suddenly were yanked from the shelves in many countries thanks to the World Trade Organisation, a branch of the United Nations, and their program of taking away supplements and over-the-counter medications. Powerful pharmaceutical companies (BigPharma) are keeping this cheap and effective remedy and hundreds more off the shelves so they can sell expensive prescriptions instead. Can you imagine needing a prescription to buy a tincture of iodine? That horrible day arrived a few years ago, and not enough people complained.

While I was working to clear toxins out of his cells, Jim consistently worked at centring, taking several deep Breaths of Life every day and listening to his *Dimensional Healing* CD. He was really an ideal client — enthusiastic and determined to get well and to keep his mood positive.

As I gradually removed toxins, his rash receded and intensity of the itching decreased. During the time we worked together, I also tightened up his bladder, got rid of an infection in his prostate and a small kidney stone. I cleared his sinuses, rebalanced his eyes, which had ceased working in harmony, and drained the fluid from his brain. His pituitary gland became very happy as his blood became clean and his circulation improved.

An added bonus from my work, was his increased

perception and awareness as his field became highly energised from head to foot. So energised, in fact, that he literally gave off sparks when he touched people. For awhile, he had to stand away from the control panel on elevators, as unpredictable things, like missing floors, would occur if he stood too close. I told him some of my own stories of shorting out electrical systems and we had a good laugh about his becoming like me.

• • • •

One day I received a distressing call from Sarah, who could barely talk through her tears. "Robyn, please help. Megan, my cat, was run over by a car. The vet said there is no hope. He's pushing me to have her put down."

"Take her home Sarah, I'll do my best." I knew what Sarah was feeling, it had happened to a dog I loved.

Sarah had owned Megan for seventeen years, since she was a six-week-old kitten. As they were leaving for work, Sarah and her partner made sure that Megan was nowhere near the driveway, but she somehow got under the wheels of the car and Sarah's partner ran over her pelvis. He was only going 3-4 miles per hour, but the cat's pelvis, directly under the wheel, was crushed.

Heartsick, they took Megan directly to the vet. An X-ray confirmed that she had a broken pelvis that left her spine twisted so that she could not pass urine or a stool. It would not be easy to operate on because of her age.

The next day the vet asked Sarah to come in. He proceeded to urge her to let the cat go. Megan was in pain, her quality of life was severely compromised, and she'd never recover from her injuries. Sarah told me that when she finally agreed to have her put to sleep, "a sudden rain poured from the sky and it went very dark. I knew it was a sign that I had made the wrong decision. I told the vet I needed another day, and just then the sun came out again."

Sarah went home and called me. I was able to link into the cat through a photograph in Sarah's house and also through her visualising her cat while we talked. I focused on getting Megan's spine straightened out and her pelvis back into the correct position. The next morning the vet told Sarah to come and get her cat. She had had a bowel movement, was more alert, and probably out of the woods.

Later, Sarah reported that Megan was eating properly, used her litter box with no problem, and was able to run up and down stairs. She drags one leg on the side where her hip was crushed, but she shows no sign of pain and is enjoying her kitty life.

Often, when I'm on the phone with clients, their pets seem to know we're in session and come running to sit next to their owner. Dogs can exhibit amazing determination to have me work with them. The dog's power can be strong enough to interrupt my concentration as I'm working on the client. This has happened a number of times. On several occasions, dogs who were locked outside two floors down barked furiously to get my attention. In one, I found a serious bowel blockage. He had obviously been in pain for some time.

• • • •

Recently a lovely woman named Caroline contacted me for help. Fifteen years earlier, she had decided to have her amalgam fillings replaced. Unfortunately, her dentist allowed mercury to escape into her body where it had been wreaking havoc with her health. By now she was so weak she was bedridden, lacking energy to perform the simplest day-to-day tasks.

"Can you get me out of this bed?" she asked.

"I'm not sure, I will have to work with you a little to see how much damage the mercury has done to your tissue and nerves."

I always try to be honest and not make false promises, so after I scanned her, I had to report that I didn't believe there were enough healthy tissues left in her body for me to do much with. Her nervous system had too many dead nerves. I would try but could make no promises. It breaks my heart when people want miracles. I really want to wave a magic wand and make it all okay!

When our sessions began, her organs responded well and began to strengthen. It was better than I had hoped.

"I have to get her out of that bed," I kept telling myself.

196

But there was a marked lack of supporting muscle tone after fifteen years of inactivity.

Caroline's husband and two sons, whom she adores, were tapped out emotionally and both had their own physical problems. They were just not able to give her the time and attention she needed. A caregiver came in, but she was essentially stranded in her house.

How would that feel? I have always been able to put myself in the other person's shoes, to empathise with them. Caroline had to depend on others for everything. Her helplessness was palpable. No matter how strong you may be, sitting up and waiting for someone to do even the smallest thing for you feels dreadful.

"Caroline," I said, "do you know of a big strong chap who will come in a few times a week to get you on your feet?" I already had her doing exercises in bed.

"Maybe my caregiver's son Joe would, he's big and strong."

"Good, get him," I said, "you are going to start dancing."

The body part that stressed Caroline the most was her bowel because she had no feeling of it when it decided to move. I went through the pain she experienced trying to have mental control over it, especially on important occasions like her son's graduation. She could not relax and enjoy outings for fear of messing herself.

Caroline's mental fear and attitude of hatred toward

it confused "Billy Bowel" to no end. In some sessions, Caroline would break down and cry, as she told me of another shocking mess in her life.

I not only had to get her out of bed, I had to strengthen her bowel, create regularity, and turn her thinking around to love it. I expended a lot of energy working with her. Joe started to come to her house three times a week. A whopping six feet and five inches tall, he had no trouble holding her rag doll body in dance position and whirling her around her room, moving her limbs as they danced. Her bowel started to strengthen and things were looking up for Caroline. I felt great admiration for her.

Just as improvements were coming about, her son was diagnosed with a heart problem that would prevent him from returning to his position as captain of the university football team. His scholarship funds and education were in jeopardy. After I worked with him for a while, his aorta went back to normal functioning and his life was back on track.

Not long afterward, Caroline's husband's colon began to bleed. Was it cancer? Don became my client and I saw that he had bleeding hemorrhoids, not cancer. I was able to fix it up for him.

Then came a financial crisis in their home. Caroline felt she had to subject herself to conventional medical treatment in order to get more support from the government.

We took a break. Months later she called broken hearted.

She had not been able to follow her doctor's advice, as it hadn't seemed right to her. They'd suggested chemo even though she didn't have cancer and her body had lost the strength it developed while we were working together. To make matters worse, Joe was not able to come any more to move her around. Her health was in trouble, her life was falling apart, and she was confined to her wheelchair.

The only bright spot in Caroline's life was her dog, Beauty, which she'd recently acquired. If she had not had Beauty, she might have been suicidal, she was so depressed and at the end of her rope. I heard the anguish in her voice when she said, "I don't have a life, why am I living?"

An idea popped into my head. "Do you live near a retirement village or an elder care village?"

"Yes," she said, "there is one just around the corner."

"Okay, here's the plan. This will be your purpose. We now know that elderly people respond well if they hug or pat a dog. Many care centres are scheduling visits from therapy pets as long as they are clean and well behaved."

The pieces began to fall into place for a wonderful new avenue for Caroline. She trained Beauty not to jump on people and found a mobile dog shampoo service to come at regular intervals to keep Beauty shiny clean. Before long, Caroline and Beauty were ready to begin visiting elderly people twice a week.

Caroline was delighted to see the good effect their visits had on the residents. Dogs have an unconditional love vibration that people feel. When they touch their soft fur their hearts rev, giving a boost to the vibrational level of their fields. Their bodies experience a surge of well being. Their health may experience a boost.

The old adage is perfectly true: "When people touch an animal, the animal touches their heart."

Nothing will make Caroline better, but her mental state has improved considerably. Beauty seems to know exactly the effect she is having on her owner. She has lifted her spirits and made her life seem worthwhile again.

• • • •

The Guide Dog Association newsletter stood out from a pile of mail one morning and I picked it up and read it first. They were offering an eight-day horse trek in the Canadian Rockies. Participants had to pay 2,500 pounds sterling to the club, which would cover expenses and a sizable donation to the organisation. I raised the money by giving sessions to clients and asking them to donate.

I'd need to get back in the saddle before leaving London, as it had been seven years since I'd done any serious riding. I went to the stable in Hyde Park and rode nice horses around the park. I should really have been better prepared, as a few days of cantering about on flat land was nowhere near enough to get my riding muscles in shape.

I left a few days ahead of the rest of the group in order to reconnect with some old friends in Seattle. While there

I gave a complimentary talk to a group as well. I then flew to Vancouver and had some time to take a look around before the other riders from London arrived for our trek. I found it to be a beautiful and exciting city with every natural and cultural advantage. I had no idea at the time that Vancouver would figure so prominently in my future, but seeds were planted. I have given up making plans; it seems God always surprises me.

The other riders arrived, all British, ranging in age from fifteen years to seventy. Most were women. I hired a sleeping bag, water bottle, torch and a few other necessities from an outback store. The rancher who supplied the horses also supplied the tents. To my delight the other riders had paired up on the flight over, so I was able to have a tent to myself. No need to clear up anyone else's frequencies, thank goodness.

That night, the group leader gave a pre-trek talk, warning that once we started the only way out was by helicopter. They would be taking our gear from base to base during the six days of actual riding. We were warned that bears were everywhere. To keep them out of our tents, we were to hand in anything pertaining to foodstuffs at the end of the day — even our toothpaste — to be placed in heavy timber boxes high up in a tree. We were warned of aggressive moose also.

We went to the barn to select our mounts. I chose Barney, a 15.2-hand grey part Percheron. His arthritis wasn't apparent on flat ground at the ranch, but I should have known that he needed healing. We set off at last, accompanied by a guide, two other men who led packhorses laden with our equipment and two talented cooks who handled some other chores as well. They all had huge rifles accessible and ready for action. Just like in the movies, I thought, "Ride 'em cowboy!"

I have to admit that our first day was the longest I have ever known. We crossed raging rivers, traversed landslides of round pebbles on slippery 14-inch wide paths that hadn't been there until the lead horses created them. Amazing horses! Severe pain took hold of me and didn't let up. My old back injuries thought they were back in hospital. After four hours in the saddle, the lunch stop was bliss. But my legs took the entire hour to work, as numbness had set in big time.

By mid afternoon, shock and searing body pain was setting into many riders, myself included. I broke into a cold sweat and my blood pressure dropped. I don't know how I stayed on Barney. It was too much to expect for the first day, and the fifteen-year-old was in a wretched state. Her mum thought they'd have to call for the helicopter to take them back to the city.

When we finally reached our overnight campsite, I could hardly dismount. I had no idea that I had legs to stand on, they were so numb. I received a quick lesson in putting up tents, and managed to secure mine satisfactorily. After a wonderful dinner, we were all ready to say goodnight. Toothpaste up in the tree, time to sleep. The horses were let loose with big bells around their necks to keep away the bears. Wolves howled their serenade. I should have slept like a baby in my 20-degrees-below sleeping bag, but I was freezing. I think they had made a mistake and given me a summer one instead.

The next day, darling Barney went into detox. As his arthritis stiffness surfaced, he sweated profusely. I'm not sure which one of us was in more pain. During the grueling eight-hour ride on day three, I kept reminding myself it was for charity and tried to work through my pain. Nothing worked.

I felt as though we were riding up and down every rugged mountain in Canada. Highly stressful, as one slip and you'd be in the raging river 200 feet below. By now my right kidney was severely bruised from Barney's pronounced rolling gait. By the fourth day, I was sure I'd lost my mind to even consider this trip. To salvage some shred of self-respect, I made up my mind that I would take my own saddle off at the end of the day like a true horseman.

I tied Barney to the rail, undid the girth, worked my arm under the saddle and three thick blankets heavy with sweat, gave an almighty heave and fell straight to the ground, saddle and all the blankets on top of me. I had only ridden in English dressage saddles previously and had no idea that the American western saddle must have been made for weightlifters.

And so we climbed and climbed to 7000 feet into a glacier, then descended Canada's most vertical drop 3000 feet in two kilometers. It was beautiful beyond the telling. God does incredible work. I thanked God I had seen it through. Another positive aspect of this experience was the water we drank from the rivers, so sweet and pure. It made me realise how bland plastic-bottled water is.

By the last day, Barney and I were moving along much better. My body was by then conditioned and he had ridded the acids from his body. We'd had our moments, but parted very good friends.

The hotel that night seemed like heaven, with a hot shower, a comfortable bed covered by crisp white sheets, a soft pillow under my head. Sweet bliss! I felt very blessed. How soft we have become. A mere hundred years ago, horses were still our main conveyance.

On arrival back in London, I threw a party to honour comfort. Having a jolly time helped my bruised and still aching body. A friend brought along a scriptwriter who worked in the film industry. As it turned out, he lived and worked in Vancouver, so we had quite a lot to talk about.

Some wonderful healings took place after my return from this challenging trip. It must have been my expanded effort of energy that boosted me to the Seventh Dimension.

Chapter Eleven
Suddenly, Vancouver

My lovely apartment in London was never meant to last forever, and all too soon the day came when the owners wanted to sell. I wasn't sure where I wanted to be. I loved London but had felt drawn to Vancouver on my last visit. It had wonderful energy and I would be able to work with the screenwriter attempting to write a movie based on *Conversations with the Body*.

Every week the people in Vancouver participate in very positive events such as walks and runs to benefit worthy causes, bike rides for various charities, religious fairs, jazz festivals and more. Never-ending celebrations are great fun and produce strong energy. The city is one of the most beautiful in the world, surrounded by mountains for skiing, beaches for swimming in the summer, and water everywhere. Vancouver has the largest city park in the world, Stanley Park, with 1000 acres of nature to roam about.

The advantages Vancouver offered far outweighed the problems of moving and off I went to make it my next home. I planned to rent a furnished apartment to try it out for a while, little knowing how difficult it was to find anything suitable to rent furnished. While looking for the right place, I stayed at a hotel I'd stayed in briefly before my horseback trek through the mountains. The desk clerk told me, "We can only put you up until Saturday, as we then have a large company conference group coming in." The pressure was on, but fortunately they found room for me for a few extra days.

Two rental ads in Saturday's newspaper sounded good. They were near the park where I wanted to be. Trouble was, they were both unfurnished. I still had a little furniture in storage in Seattle, just over the border. It couldn't be too difficult to bring it up, could it? I could purchase a few more things I'd need.

I didn't love the first apartment I viewed and couldn't find the other. In my desperation, I was almost ready to sign a lease but I decided to take a break. I sat in a coffee bar to think about the apartment I'd seen. The price was good and the interior designer in me could jazz it up. Then the deeper thought dropped in, Robyn, the other apartment is nearby, ask directions from the cashier on the way out. "It's just two blocks away," she said.

When I saw the apartment, I loved it. It had been completely refurbished, the water view was stunning, and it rented for less than the other one. I was very excited. Now all I needed was to have my furniture brought up from storage in Seattle.

I zipped around Vancouver buying a few things I'd need and made arrangements with a friend in Seattle to drive my things up in a van. There was one huge logistical problem to solve, however. In a single day, I had to be at the United States/Canadian border, two and a half hours away if traffic is flowing and also had be at the apartment to accept delivery of a bed and pick up my keys from the apartment manager.

My friend Nick from Seattle came up to help. We drove down to the border to meet the moving van containing my household goods, which had to be inspected before it could come through. Nick got lost on the way because he spaced out in an altered state in my company and took an hour longer than necessary. The inconvenient truth is that I have this effect on people I come in contact with. If I talk with people who are driving me around, even taxi drivers, they tend to space out. It only occurs if they need healing, and almost everyone does now.

The truck was waiting for us when we arrived, but the driver's helper was not allowed to enter Canada, as his paperwork was not up to scratch. I told Nick to go back to Seattle and take the helpless helper with him. I sat next to the driver in the truck and made my grand entrance into Vancouver. It was shake, rattle and roll all the way. We finally reached the apartment where two men who would help unload met us. The driver had arranged for them while waiting for me at the border.

All of my goods were packed in big cardboard boxes — even large pieces of furniture. I hadn't realised that the wrapping had a tar base for waterproofing. I made an arrangement for a handyman to help me flatten the huge heavy boxes and take them to the basement twenty-four floors below, jobs I thought beyond me. But he couldn't come until Monday. Impatient, I began the enormous job of unpacking on my own. My lounge room became a jumble of cardboard boxes and wrapping and I became increasingly nauseous and weak from the chemicals the tarpaper gave off. By Sunday night, I realised the poison problem. "Don't worry Robyn," I told myself, "Jack the handyman will be here in the morning."

Monday came and went and Jack did not show up. To add to my woes, my phone was still not connected. I flopped down dejected and ill. You have to do it yourself, you have to clear it out of your space, or you'll die. To this day, I don't know how I managed that heavy lifting and carrying. (I keep saying I don't know where I find the energy, but actually I do.)

After getting all the boxes to the basement, I took a rest on my balcony, gulping fresh air into my grateful lungs. I gathered some blankets to rug up against the chill of late winter and took in my wonderful view. Out on the water, lovely sailboats picked up the early evening breeze to glide toward the deep blue water of the bay. My mind drifted back to my childhood home when I would lie in the lush green grass of the pasture and stare into the sky after my mother's death, hoping to see her face implanted in the sky where I thought heaven was located.

I slept deeply and awoke to see the sunrise on distant mountaintops still covered with deep snow sure to delight skiers and other winter sports enthusiasts. I began to sense that I wasn't alone in my bedroom. As I alighted from my bed two pigeons scattered. Obviously they had entered through my open window. "Shoo, go out," I gently told them, but they were in no hurry to leave.

That night I made sure my window was only partly open, so they won't be able to come in again. The next morning, much to my surprise, there they were. They'd managed to get in again. This time I was a little firmer in my request that they leave, as one or both had left a calling card on my spare pillow. For a week I slept with the windows shut.

The next week, I discovered that one of the pigeons had made a nest tucked away in a corner of the balcony. She was quite comfortable with my presence; she didn't even attempt to fly away. Apparently the pair had tried to nest in my bedroom. They wanted a human nursery for their two eggs to hatch in. So once again, wild pets had come into my life to bring me joy.

I checked the nest every few days and one day was horrified to see a hatchling that had somehow separated from the warmth of its mother. It was freezing cold and looked dead, but I picked it up, gave it healing energy, and life appeared again. I quietly approached its mother who actually allowed me to tuck it back under her. It grew into a fine bird, as did the other. I believe the pigeons were sent to me as karma for the anguish I suffered one freezing night in Seattle, and the lessons I learned about myself.

Many Pigeons in the City

Peak hour evening bus rush, freezing conditions
Red cold bodies, waiting at the stop
Anxious to return to warm abodes
To re-energise for the next workday

No one seemed to notice or care
About the old pigeon, obviously very ill
No doubt facing his last hours of life
Still trying to survive as always

Different now, no longer proud steps
That he had always taken, chest out
Moving among the travellers waiting
For life-giving crumbs, to be dropped

Instead, now staggering, faulty steps
Taken slowly, before gasping for air
One wing spread, for ground support

Still hoping for a life-giving crumb

I feel so useless, to help ease his pain
Bus close by and only fare money
Shop nearby, full of wonderful crumbs
Should I go in and beg some?

No I am too proud and embarrassed
I can only pray that his end is swift
As I catch the 206 tears in my eyes
I sit down with many thoughts and feelings
What use was I to this poor creature?
No use because of pride to ask
Which is no sin, for many have to do so
I see city streets full of them

I also notice, that most do not notice
These street-people, who like the pigeon
Survival depending on sharing and kindness
From the passing strong ones

I felt such remorse on that bus
For myself, the pigeon and the street-people
For the weakness and the suffering
During the Christmas season of '95.

Robyn Elizabeth Welch

••••

Vancouver was to become my graduate school, as Seattle had been my university years earlier. By the end of 2005, I knew I had entered the Ninth Dimension, I had no need to do my breathing exercises or play my clock games anymore, I instinctively knew I was there. I have been strengthened to cope with every new event in this journey, to heal every new soul who energetically reaches out for my help. I experienced lengthy spells of exhaustion as I was being conditioned to cope with my increasing responsibilities. I'd get so tired I'd have to remind myself that this is what I'd prayed for so long ago when I'd asked God if I was intended to heal others.

In London, many thousands of new people learned about me. Within a short period of time my book was published, my web site went up, and my CD was released. Exhaustion set in and it took me some time to figure out the reason. Finally I realised that my heartbeat was running for 60 seconds in the sample of my CD on my web site and people from all over the world who were seeking healing were plugging into it. I was pleased that so many people were finding me online, but I was feeling the pull. Cutting back to 15 seconds of heartbeat made a big improvement in my personal energy level. I'd been expending healing energy to everyone listening to my heartbeat. I'm running on automatic now; it just happens.

I have to go to movies on weekday afternoons to avoid crowds. I sit as far away from other moviegoers but even so, I cannot escape. I clean negative frequencies from the theatre and the audience. People have their mobile phones with them, so that makes extra work for me. Even if they are turned off, the frequencies they put out can be damaging. Theatres, restaurants, markets — every new space I enter engages my healing skills. For this reason, I seldom go out. But the world was coming to me.

By the time I moved to Vancouver, my CD had been out for two years, and I was getting enthusiastic thanks from people who used it. For a long time I had dreamed of a small handheld device that would contain my work. Then the personal music player (PMP) burst onto the market. It stores ten hours of play, once charged, and can be taken anywhere. It was so ideal, it seemed inventors might have developed it just for me.

I wrote a script and went to a recording studio. I'd learned a lot from my experience in the London studio so I was in and out of the Vancouver studio before all of the negative frequencies of electronic instruments affected me too much. I was very pleased with the resulting PMP with nothing but my recorded messages and vibrations on it. Jennifer Hunter, an Australian physician, had tested my CD and discovered that the purity of the vibration is ruined by computer play or downloading from a computer. Therefore, I instruct those who obtain my PMPs not to download anything else on it. If they do so, its healing potential is compromised, defeating the purpose of owning it.

My PMP is getting rave reviews. Clients tell me that it's a tremendous help in clearing negative frequencies from their fields, thereby maintaining their positive energy. A few people reported that they'd taken my PMP on airplane trips and reached their destinations feeling refreshed and energetic. What a good idea. I tried it out on an international flight and it helped keep my energy strong during the long flight in spite of miles of wiring and electronic instruments on the jet. I won't leave home without it again. Actually, I'm delighted to have found a way to used technology in a positive, helpful way.

While I'll have more pulls and tugs on my energy from those who use my CD and PMP, my increasing ability to rise to higher dimensions more than balances the load. As my consciousness opens out to new dimensions, my sessions become more powerful and I'm able to access more information. I have no doubt that every positive word spoken is recorded in what mystics call the Akashic Records in the form of electrical frequencies. Negative frequencies survive if locked into natural material; positive frequencies live on forever.

As I became established in the higher dimension, I wanted more answers. I knew that half of my work was spiritual and that my heart generates the driving force behind the energy ray. But what about the other 50 percent of my work? Where was this energy zone I was using for healings? I have always questioned, always tried to work things out using common sense and logical thinking. But still, I didn't have the answers to how I could manipulate the body in sessions; why was so-called matter like putty in my hands?

I found good information in the work of George Lakhovsky, a Russian bioengineer whose book, *Secret of Life*, published in 1925, fits into today's knowledge. There is no doubt whatsoever that we are vibrating electrical beings running on positive and negative energy.

Dr Lakhovsky believed that when body cells are at war it's a radiation war. If the radiation of the microbe wins, disease and death are imminent. If the cell's own positive transmission wins, health is preserved. I agree with this theory. Albert Nodan, President of Astronomique of Bordeaux was able to prove Lakhovsky's hypothesis.

Lakhovsky made wonderful discoveries concerning our two hundred thousand trillion cells and our DNA molecules. His discoveries were corroborated by Roger Coghill a distinguished British research scientist. Lakhovsky proved that a living cell could be compared to an electrical oscillating circuit. This nucleus consists of tubular filaments, chromosomes and mitochondria, made of insulating membranes, but filled by an electrically conductive and inductance properties.

Cells are capable of working like radio transmitters sending and receiving. My theory to add to his is that this energy runs clockwise from our cells. Roger Coghill went a step further to add that glyco-proteins, which are sugary molecules, stand up from the cell surface to act like little aerials. I believe that every cell in our bodies is sending and receiving energy every second of the day.

Still, I had questions about where my work fit into the great search for universal answers.

Conversations With Einstein

It was time to turn to the master of matter and energy, Albert Einstein. I'd long been an admirer and cherished some of the things he'd said: "Problems can not be solved at the same level of awareness that created them." "The philosophy of one generation is commonsense to the next."

I went to the bookstore and brought home some of Einstein's books, hoping to find enlightenment. I wanted to go further than his theory $E = mc^2$. Energy equals matter times the speed of light squared. I was fascinated that at some velocity, energy equals matter. In my work, energy certainly changes matter, so Einstein's work felt right to me — though of course his complex equations were far beyond my grasp. A physics professor had told me that I had to be travelling faster than the speed of light to do the work I do. That made sense, as I knew that light takes eight minutes to travel from the sun to Earth. We can send thoughts there in a fraction of that time.

Since Einstein, we have learned that subatomic particles can communicate and affect each other instantaneously, even if they have been separated to opposite ends of the universe. Particles can flip in and out of existence as they move between matter and anti-matter. Depending on how you view electrons, they will behave like a light wave or a solid particle. So, all in all, rules that apply in everyday life do not apply to the subatomic world.

While I cannot prove it with mathematics, I know that when I am in session, I move my energy and my client's body parts into a space where light stands still. There seems to be no difference, no line of demarcation between the vast sea of light and the atoms and cells of the body. In the three dimensional world, there are observable differences, but they disappear in the highest dimensions where my consciousness can use energy to make changes in ailing bodies that are, in that moment of time and space, part of the larger energy. As is my consciousness. In this amazing beautiful space, all is possible.

Wanting to know all I could about this amazing place, I reached out to Einstein, "Where are you?" I swear I felt his presence here on my lounge, right where I'm sitting now, for one week. I took in new information and some that confirmed my experiential knowledge. I came to know that the amazing place is a space, a dimension, although not large. Step out of this space and you're in heaven. This is the zone I levitate my bodies to for healing. (It may be the doorway to Heaven.) Here the behaviour of atoms, particles, light and energy can be observed. Energy and matter are the same. Depending on how you view electrons in this quantum world, a force field only appears to fill all space smoothly and continuously.

Examined closely, light consists of tiny packets of energy called quanta or photons. They can behave like a light wave or a solid particle. Rules that seem to apply to everyday life don't apply to the subatomic world. Here, matter is converted to energy by splitting the atom that releases the enormous energy stored within the nucleus.

Now here is where this mind-blowing information really became interesting. Jesus did not actually die; he appeared to be dead with nothing functioning in his body. He went to this quantum zone, healed and returned to earth.

I was informed that I had been there also. I remember nothing of this visit. However, this information did fit into readings done by three leading clairvoyants who told me that I had died in the car accident in 1981 and crossed to the other side. Not one of them had known I'd been in an accident or anything else about me. But going to the quantum zone and back would explain how I get there so easily now, rather like a homing pigeon. I believe that many others have been there, which would explain the scratches found on the inside of coffin lids when bodies are exhumed.

From further information relayed to me, this kickstart of a body would happen only if a person has a strong energy field during their lifetime and a heart that has not been physically destroyed at time of death. I'm asking my family to delay my burial for five days.

I'm happy with the information I received. It makes sense to me that the power to ascend to higher dimensions comes from our energy field and magnetic forces. There are no safety nets for this flight, no earthly security blankets. I share this with you, knowing of the disbelief that will come from many with a cynical viewpoint, who find it impossible to believe my work, let alone my conversation with Einstein.

The quantum zone is indeed a truly Divine place. Here there is no ownership, no money, no possessions, just pure joy, happiness and Divine love. It's as close as we can get to heaven on earth. It's going to become easier for many because our knowledge is increasing and our DNA is changing. We're in the midst of an accelerated period of evolvement and advancement of consciousness. This is the time for people on earth to connect to this zone where all positive things are possible. Will the future be positive or negative? The choice is in our hands.

Yes, God can move mountains. But what about people? Can we be the cause of natural events too? I awoke one morning to the newscaster saying that a major earthquake was expected to hit over the weekend under Victoria, the beautiful capitol city of British Columbia located on nearby Vancouver Island. If Victoria shook, so would Vancouver and we have taller buildings. I decided to see whether I could do anything to avert the calamity. As I've mentioned, in higher dimensions, nothing exists but love. Why not send huge amounts of love to the tectonic plates threatening to shift under Victoria? Perhaps that would relieve some stress and help drain negative frequencies from this impending explosion. I visualised, I smoothed out underground cracks, I gently swept the ground with my ray, spreading soft loving energy all over the threatened island. Next morning I awake to learn that no quake had occurred. Nor on the next.

Our huge earthquake never happened. I have no way to know whether my work actually helped or how many other good people prayed too.

Polar Bear Swim

On New Years Day, 2007, a large polar bear swim was scheduled at English Bay, right downstairs from my apartment. I hadn't had a challenge since the Canadian Mountain Horseback Ride, so decided to sign up. I'd always been interested in what goes on in the human body exposed to freezing temperatures. I became very excited about the swim and prepared myself mentally, which is difficult for something you've never experienced.

Two thousand bold and possibly crazy swimmers

showed up, some still intoxicated from the night before. As I stood in the midst of the crowd, I wondered how their numbed bodies would handle the freezing temperatures. There could be many casualties, I supposed.

I clung to my layers of warm clothing until the go signal. It seemed to take an age to push through those hundreds who had run into the water up to the waist, then turned around screaming for shore. I proceeded into the water at a steady pace. At last at waist level, I dove in and started swimming straight out. Shocking! I tried to breathe as my body temperature rapidly declined. Getting control over my reaction, I settled into a steady stroke, willing myself to get used to the frigid water. By now I was well away from shore. I stopped and rolled onto my back. I could see that there were about twenty swimmers left in the water. It was then that I felt my body change, as though all my nerves were jumping. Better head back now.

I started stroking freestyle. A feeling of heaviness was overtaking my body and I began to feel somewhat disoriented. With that came a panicky feeling, something I'm not used to. Will my feet ever touch the sand? After what seemed an eternity, there it was. I'd made it!

On my way to collect my badge, I noticed some swimmers collapsing, their bodies limp as rag dolls. They looked very uncomfortable. My clothing started to restore my icy body. It took ages to warm up. I proudly viewed my award thinking I would not have missed the experience for anything. Something else I experienced firsthand about the body that night: I sent warm love through it and once again thanked it for teaching me something else about the amazing human system.

Chapter Twelve
Accessing Higher Dimensions

Over the years I had frequently heard of other dimensions, but had never really experienced such things until I had meditated for several years and gradually found myself moving into higher dimensions.

The intense energy frequencies I experienced in those spaces enabled me to do finer, more meticulous healing work. In fact, my progression into higher dimensions often occurred spontaneously when I needed more power, vision, and strength to heal a difficult case. The work itself became the vehicle that took me to higher dimensions.

Students who attended my healing classes asked how they could reach these higher dimensions. First of all, one must learn to view life as energy. Then, I believe that controlling your mind is the jumping off place. Your mind can either take you to heaven or dump you in hell. Anyone unable to still the mind and concentrate his or her full attention on the work will have problems learning. Cultivating a calm, steady mind is a key to healing in higher dimensions. Untrained it will not allow you to go into the still space where no earthly thing exists. This is the powerful quantum zone where all is still. We know that even Einstein's theory changes here.

Before I began teaching classes to those who wanted to learn my healing method, I gave a lot of thought to how I would transmit the knowledge that I had built up over more than two decades. More than knowledge was involved, of course. How would I be able to transmit my ability to see inside the body? To speak to the body and be understood? To heal from higher dimensions of consciousness? I believed I'd be able to teach if those signing up for the classes were prepared to allow the work to develop gradually in their lives. The process required time and a certain amount of sacrifice so that their evolution could reach to higher dimensions.

I arranged for space and began to teach the twenty-five people who'd signed up. It was disappointing for me, as only two showed any real promise of becoming effective healers. The others wanted to learn overnight, hoping to attend one class and work to my standard. Some admitted that the process I'd gone through frightened them. They did not want to make any sacrifices to attain proficiency in this finely tuned healing method. They were unrealistic.

I cannot overstress the fact that healing is demanding work that requires much from practitioners.

In my experience, those who are able to learn begin with a certain innate talent, which many people have, combined with strong willpower and a burning desire to heal. Humility is an important attribute that helps them put aside preconceived notions and open themselves to learning. Ideally, healers should make their minds keen, their focus sharp, their hearts strong and their bodies radiantly healthy... and keep their egos out of the way. Of course, they need psychic sensitivity to perceive the infinite subtleties of the body and its energy.

I looked for students with dedication, determination, unwavering desire, and purity of intention. Self-discipline is indispensable. Healing requires gentleness as well as sound bodies and minds. And patience, caring, kindliness, compassion, and love, love, love. I cannot imagine healers succeeding who lack a spiritual connection to a higher power, call it what they will.

That's admittedly an extensive list. I can always hope for the ideal student but he or she is probably a figment of my imagination. However, anyone I teach should be prepared to develop all the qualities I've mentioned. When healing and when rising to higher dimensions, you'll need to draw on these strengths. I now believe that teaching will be more successful by attaching them to my frequency.

Quieting the Mind

It's hard to achieve a quiet mind because day-to-day stress, overexposure to the constant din of media, and the endless assault by inharmonious frequencies drain our energy and dump us into the fourth dimension, a dark void above our three earthly dimensions, where impossibilities live. As much as I enjoy the practice of meditation, I caution you to approach it carefully.

Meditation taught by trustworthy gurus and other reliable teachers gets us attuned to at least the fifth dimension, where love and compassion dwell. Do not meditate with an untrained mind because you probably will not have enough electrical strength to tune you into the higher vibrations or dimensions. You have to learn how to establish yourself in a higher vibrational state to keep from burning out — that's the power required to connect you to real spiritual dimensions.

You need laser-like focus to advance beyond the ordinary third dimension world we live in, boost yourself over the negative fourth dimension, and attune to the fifth and beyond. Unless your mind is absolutely still during meditation, you are wasting your time and possibly inviting negativity into your life. We now know that the brain is electrical, and if it is allowed to overwork, it tires of power to hold higher dimensions so crashes into negative dimensions.

Still Your Mind for Thirty Seconds

Here is the best exercise I've ever found to get your mind ready for meditation and healing. Set aside time to practise this exercise two or three times daily.

Sit in a comfortable place.

Place a clock or watch with a second hand where you can see it without strain.

Resolve to keep your mind quiet for 30 seconds.

Take the Breath of Life — inhale deeply, hold for eight seconds, and exhale through rounded lips.

Close your eyes and communicate with your mind saying, "Mind I love you and need you but for now go over there and be still."

Empty your mind. Be adamant with your message, especially during early training or your mind will easily overpower you.

It may take a long time to achieve your 30-second goal. Be persistent and eventually you'll get there. As you gradually progress beyond the thirty-second mark, you will find that you will get into a meditative state more easily, almost automatically. You'll move into the bliss and joy of true spirituality where all knowledge lies. Once you're anchored to these higher zones in meditation you will remain there, whether or not thoughts come into your mind.

Tune Your Mind to Higher Dimensions

On a trip to Hawaii to give a seminar, I discovered another useful method for working with the mind. I was lying on the beach when I had an idea that would help with my teaching. Again, the visualisation was a clock. This one would help me tune my vibration to the Divine energy.

In my visualisation I placed a clock just above my head. I designated twelve o'clock as God's radio station. If I could get both hands to point to twelve, I'd know I was perfectly attuned to the Divine.

My first attempt put me at 11:50. Not bad for starters, but I wanted to be perfectly tuned. I knew what I needed to do. I was able to jiggle every cell in my body, thereby moving the big hand to the twelve o'clock position. I enjoyed my new game and was delighted to have discovered a method for making sure I'm perfectly in vibration with the fifth dimension.

Next day, I couldn't wait to play my game again. This time, I was at 11:58, much better than yesterday, I thought. So I did my jiggling act, which started to take me above the twelve o'clock. This unnerved me for some reason. Come back to the clock, I told myself, feeling that it was my safety zone.

Next day, I was above the clock from the start. My deep thought told me that it was okay. "Robyn let go and soar." The penny dropped so to speak and I knew I was in the sixth dimension. As with every climb I would experience, this led to evolvement not only in my work but also in my awareness and knowledge.

I was given this exercise to demonstrate that I was ready to soar into the sixth dimension. Previously, I hadn't even known there were more than five dimensions. I wanted to know I was perfectly attuned to God's radio station but instead I was shown there were more dimensions to rise through.

I hoped for further development and eagerly awaited another manifestation of spirit that would advance me to the next stage of evolvement. I didn't have to wait long. It was revealed on a subsequent trip to Hawaii, the magnificent part of the world that has been so significant to my journey.

One evening on Oahu, I sat in the outdoor restaurant of a pretty pink hotel right on the beach. I'd ordered dinner and was gazing at the beauty of the sun setting over the ocean waiting for my meal to be served. Far out in the water, I saw two people up to their necks awkwardly supporting something between them, Oh no! I thought a boat had hit a turtle and injured it. It seemed an eternity for this man and woman to reach shallow water. As they approached the beach, I saw that they were dragging the body of a woman between them.

Without even thinking, I kicked off my shoes, jumped the four-foot chain onto the sand and sprinted toward them. The couple that had dragged her in were Japanese and could not communicate in English with the four men who had gathered on the sand. No one was doing anything but looking down with alarm at the unconscious woman "Quickly, go get help!" I yelled at them. I immediately sank to my knees in the wet sand, cleared her open mouth and began mouth-to-mouth resuscitation. Without even wondering why, I worked on her heart at the same time.

With great relief, I heard her start to breathe. "It's okay," I told her gently, "you will be okay now." The woman started to cry and was mumbling incoherently. A peculiar reaction. Had she tried to commit suicide?

"Don't cry," I said, as reassuringly as possible.

"You don't understand," she cried, "I need aspirin, I recently had heart surgery."

"Get aspirin someone!" I yelled, still soothing her, although knowing instinctively that she would not need it. "Here come the paramedics," I said, "they will take you for a good check-up."

"I don't need them," she said, "I'm feeling fine." Quite a difference from the comatose woman she'd been ten minutes earlier.

A female paramedic yelled at the poor woman to stand up, expecting her to walk 200 yards across the heavy sand to the roadside where the ambulance was parked.

I was thoroughly disgusted with her intimidating attitude. "Look here," I yelled, "this woman has just had a near death experience, leave her alone you bully. And why didn't you bring a stretcher?"

I was by then standing toe to toe with her. "Who are you anyway?" she commanded, with her I've-had-a-bad-day voice.

"She is the person who brought me back to life," the

woman said, hugging me and crying again. "Thank you, thank you. What's your name?"

"Robyn," I said, "go with the paramedics, they will want to check you out."

As I turned to go back up the beach to the restaurant, I saw hundreds of people who had collected to watch the drama. As I approached they cheered, "Well done, good on you!" Dinner was on the house, many beautiful leis were placed around my neck and my purse was still on the table.

That night in bed, I thanked God for the opportunity to save a life. I was quite sure the woman had literally returned from the dead. The more I thought about it, the more amazed I was that I'd been part of the process. I knew I was being released from a karmic debt, as decades earlier I had not been able to revive a neighbour's baby who'd drowned in my pool. The thought so overwhelmed me, I cried tears of gratitude.

Upon waking next morning I realised the real value of my lifesaving effort, all my karmas were coming into harmony, allowing me to fly in higher dimensions.

When I returned to London, there was a stack of glowing reports waiting for me from those I had worked on by telephone. My confidence took a quantum leap forward. Each time I entered a higher dimension on this journey, my work evolved and my awareness became keener.

I no longer had to take time to get myself into the

healing zone. It was as though I were attuned to it automatically. I was instantaneously grounded and ready to go to work.

My Journey Through Higher Dimensions

I would like to take you on a journey and endeavour to explain my trip through the dimensional levels that I have experienced.

Since ancient times, mystics have been aware that other aspects, or dimensions, of reality exist that can be accessed through meditation, ritual, or other spiritual practices — and sometimes spontaneously. Integral psychologist Ken Wilber explains, wisdom traditions subscribe to the notion that reality manifests in levels or dimensions, with each higher dimension being more inclusive and therefore 'closer' to the absolute totality of Godhead or Spirit. In this sense, Spirit is the summit of being, the highest rung on the ladder of evolution."

While spiritual traditions may disagree about what higher dimensions actually mean, they generally agree about the existence of a region beyond the three earthly dimensions we think of as everyday reality. One reason they disagree, I believe, is that they cannot get beyond thinking in terms of positive or negative. Perhaps they feel it reflects badly on their authority for people to ascend to higher dimensions on their way to heaven without their leadership. But I know it is happening. This energy I'm connected with has never lied to me. Spirit does not lie. The human problem lies in the interpretation of the communication. I've been my own worst critic, at first especially, questioning everything, making sure that my impressions were true and pure.

Each and every dimension is reached from generated heart power, which tunes the human energy field into higher vibrations. Love is the only thing that works the heart generator. It is producing frequencies that come out from the bottom of the heart. Only the feeling of love can produce the frequency needed to pitch our vibration.

The higher your vibration, the greater your feelings of joy and bliss, which you reach simply because your heart is so full of love for all things. We are vibrational electrical beings. Part of the evolvement we are going through now will raise us to higher frequency levels. In a sense, we are becoming frequency beings.

The climb is now going to be easier because we have been going through an accelerated leap of consciousness. Jesus moved evolution forward by 3000 years; now, since 1994, we have been going through another boost. This time our DNA and cells are changing us rapidly as they evolve to pick up higher vibrations. Each cell has a tiny antenna that is beginning to attune to higher frequencies. Within a short time, this attunement will advance our evolution by 2000 years.

No matter how easy it is becoming, every individual

has to free themselves from attachments and bondage in order to fly. On the other hand, you cannot live there. You can only visit these glorious zones. Exploring higher dimensions is part of life, but you must not direct your full energy to it.

Many mystics and spiritual people have been aware of a shift in consciousness for years. Even in repressive Communist China, there are those with the sensitivity to feel it and the courage to speak about their new awareness. I particularly like this brilliant observation by Master li Hongzhi, leader of a large spiritual group called Falun Zuan: "If you can enter the space between cells and molecules or the spaces among molecules, you will experience being in another dimension. At that time, you will find it also a boundless dimension."

Multi-dimensional Reality

On a somewhat similar track, mathematicians and theoretical physicists have been looking at the possibility of multi-dimensional reality since the mid-1980s. They are working on superstring and membrane theories (M-theory) in hopes of developing a "unified theory of everything." Theoretical physicists hypothesise the existence of ten or eleven physical dimensions — or perhaps as many as twenty-six — that they hope will explain every phenomenon in the universe. Major universities spend millions on research and some of the best minds in physics are working on superstring theory today. But few if any scientists relate their work in any way to the intuitions of major spiritual leaders down through the ages.

We have to be very careful to avoid misinterpreting sophisticated mathematical data we don't really understand. Nevertheless, the literature about string theory written for non-physicists is full of tantalising references that sound very spiritual indeed. The most mind-boggling for me is the statement by renowned physicist Michio Kaku, Ph.D., of New York University in his excellent book *Beyond Einstein* that echoes my personal experience with higher dimensions:

"A ten-dimensional being looking down on our universe could see all of our internal organs and could even perform surgery on us without cutting our skin. This idea of reaching into a solid object without breaking the outer surface seems absurd to us only because our minds are limited when considering higher dimensions..."

Spiritual explorers are usually willing to look at scientific evidence that supports their intuitive experiences; one can only hope that scientists might take an open-minded view of experiential evidence. It's a problem for them because they cannot put feelings into numbers.

In his profound book, *The Universe In A Single Atom: The Convergence of Science and Spirituality*, His Holiness the Dalai Lama explores this idea. "Many aspects of reality as well as some key elements of human existence, such as the ability to distinguish between good and evil, spirituality, artistic creativity — some of the things we most value about human beings — inevitably fall outside the scope of the [scientific] method. Scientific knowledge, as it stands today, is not complete. ...clearly recognising the limits of scientific knowledge, I believe, is essential."

Some scientists are exploring the concept of a higher power. In *Parallel Worlds: A Journey Through Creation, Higher Dimensions, and the Future Of The Cosmos*, Michio Kaku writes, "...a miraculous set of 'accidents' makes consciousness possible in this three-dimensional universe of ours. The stability of the proton, the size of the stars, the existence of higher elements and so on, all seem to be finely tuned to allow for complex forms of life and consciousness... no one can dispute the intricate tuning necessary to make us possible.

Stephen Hawking remarks, "If the rate of expansion one second after the big bang had been smaller by even one part in a hundred thousand million, [the universe] would have recollapsed before it reached its present size... the odds against a universe like ours emerging out of something like the big bang are enormous. I think there are clearly religious implications."

Despite these glimmerings, science and spirituality still seem light-years apart. Perhaps it's because scientists are inclined to leave love out of the equation. In my work, each and every higher dimension is reached from love, the generated heart power that tunes the human energy field into higher vibrations. You might think of the climb through higher dimensions as your inner stairway to heaven.

Third Dimension

Our ordinary senses register the three dimensions of everyday reality: length, breadth and height. We live in planet Earth's three-dimensional school, a lovely place we share with animals and plants and people we love. Some people who want to go to the top of the class consider Earth as a springboard to higher dimensions. Climbing from these three dimensions into higher realms takes a huge amount of work on oneself daily to bring about a focused mind and to purify our thoughts and feeling. We must struggle to overcome the negativity of chemicals and electronic instruments we've invented to reach the beauty of our heartfelt feelings. Earth school is tough. We need to learn to tune into the patterns of beauty that uplift us.

In the third dimension, our big job is to get ready to evolve into higher dimensions. Every living thing on planet Earth dies. No one escapes. Although most don't want to think about the next part of our journey, Heaven is there, open to all who maintain positive energy. Negative energy is destructive. Beautiful Divine energy is healthy and constructive. Prayer works if you connect energetically with God. An abundance of Divine Love energy is available to all willing to put forth the effort to connect with it. We can draw on the power of this love frequency whenever we need it, especially when we need to move to a higher dimension.

Positive energy is especially significant when our adventure of this lifetime is finished. Heaven, as it's known, is the stopping off place. All the goodness you have built by endeavouring to be a positive person comes into being there, imprinted on one frequency of our soul. All of our lifetime information, including that from other lifetimes, becomes arrayed in our fields, in karmic harmony.

At the time of death, a powerful soul who has positive energy to spare is virtually rocket-thrust from the three earthly dimensions. Tremendous power is needed for this journey, enough to avoid the negative fourth dimension and connect with the fifth dimension where it absorbs very high energy to give it another boost to take it into the realms of Heaven.

We've come back to this lifetime to remove negativity from our souls. Each lifetime is another opportunity to balance our karma. Religions do a good job of encouraging us to be good people and lead clean lives. Doing so helps our energy fields accumulate enough positive energy to move us up through the dimensions. Those who do not follow the Golden Rule will have energy fields riddled with the static of electrical interference and will be stuck in the fourth dimension. I always advise people to live their lives with the intention of ascending through higher dimensions. You can fine-tune your abilities so you'll be ready to zoom into at least the fifth dimension. It helps with living in three dimensions if you can attune to higher dimensions now and then.

Fourth Dimension

The fourth dimension is hell as we know it. Old time preachers were not far off the mark describing fire and brimstone because negativity has to explode. Until it explodes, it is three times stronger than positive. I call the fourth dimension the dark land without love.

As I mentioned, certain psychics, intuitives, and spiritual leaders have tried to describe dimensional space, and scientists are now working to describe the physical version of dimensional space as well. Superstring theorists are positing ten, eleven or more dimensions to describe the fabric of reality. Their extensive tests revealed mysterious dark matter and dark energy that pervade the universe. Lisa Randall, a leading theoretical physicist working on superstring theory at Harvard writes, "Dark matter is the nonluminous matter that pervades the universe... even though about one-quarter of the energy in the universe is stored in dark matter, we still don't know what it is... The universe contains dark energy that constitutes 70% of the total energy in the universe."

Non-luminous is the perfect word to describe the fourth dimension. I cannot precisely define every aspect of the darkness of the fourth dimensional void but I believe that dark matter is collective negative frequencies. I am sure that if our personal energy field is riddled with negative interference, we'll be unable to stay out of the darkness of the fourth dimension. We must bear in mind that negative frequencies have multiplied in the past sixty years. Adding to this is the blanket of pollution weighing heavily over the entire planet. How can the human body, with millions of years of evolution behind it, suddenly cope with the massive onslaught of electromagnetic radiation it must increasingly deal with?

According to Robert O. Becker, M.D. author of the 1985 bestseller, *The Body Electric*, "Large parts of the energy spectrum were totally silent before 1883," when Thomas Edison set up the first electric-power system in New York. "We'll never experience that quiet world again... Since then, nearly every human action has involved an electrical appliance and today we're all awash in a sea of energies life has never before experienced... The human species has changed its electromagnetic background more than any other aspect of the environment."

Keep in mind that Dr Becker wrote this more than 25 years ago. Since then, the electromagnetic background we have to contend with has amped up considerably, especially since wireless mobile phones, laptops and other gadgets were invented. In the years since Becker wrote his book, we have not seen a noticeable improvement in the quality of human minds and hearts that might balance out the negativity of electromagnetic radiation. It's an incredible struggle today to keep our personal vibrations on the positive side of the ledger. Who would have believed this day would arrive when we need to shampoo negative frequencies lodged in our energy fields just as we clean our bodies and clothing.

This void is now overloaded with lost souls. I say lost souls because most lost self-control during their lifetimes — those addicted to drugs, alcohol, sex, crime and other unwholesome chemicals or processes were on a negative path, helpless to turn their lives around. Other souls are stuck in the fourth dimensional "land without love" because they intentionally treated people badly during their lifetimes, giving free rein to their own aggression, arrogance, materialism and a host of other offenses without regard for the misery they caused others. We all do unkind things, but without intent to hurt, our heart generators are still running and we don't end up in the fourth dimensions. If you do horrid things with intent, that's another story. The fourth dimension is home to untold millions of rapists, murderers, pedophiles, pornographers, thieves, sadists, cheats, and other unsavoury sorts. Believe me, you don't want to go there.

The frequencies of mobile phones can align people with this zone whether they are sending or receiving. Mobile phones operate on a range of frequencies. They

241

"roam" looking for an available frequency whenever a call is made. While roaming, they are collecting more and more power. Unfortunately they affect women more than men because we are on a higher vibrational level. Negative emotions can stem from neurological damage caused by mobile phone frequencies. Users become addicted, not to speaking with their friends but to the frequencies mobile phones emit. (How many times have you heard people say they love their mobile phones?) You may think that warm, friendly conversations would generate the heart, and they may for a short time. However, the negative power of the mobile phone overwhelms the love frequency.

Positive Helpful Frequencies

Instead of remaining addicted to mobile phone frequencies, we might just as easily become captivated by positive, helpful frequencies. At about this time, a London friend called my attention to little portable media players called PMPs and I began to experiment to see whether I could develop a way to transmit positive energy. Ideally, we could transplant loving positive frequencies into homes and working spaces to counteract negative frequencies and help people climb to higher dimensions. Finding the PMP, which plays audio, turned out to be the key, but it took me awhile before I figured out exactly what was required to get the desired result.

Some unfortunate souls have been sent to the darkness

unwittingly by trained professionals who advised them to take chemo and radiation treatment for cancer. Most of the time, these treatments do little more than bring them a Band-Aid, usually followed by more suffering with no quality of life and an undignified death. I've heard this story in every Western country. Cancer is diagnosed and surgery is recommended. The patient is told that the operation was a success: Everything was properly removed, but just to make sure, chemo or radiation is suggested. Chemo and radiation attack the patient's every cell and energy field, weakening them, causing the body to run on negative energy. At the time of death, these victims have no positive energy that would help them avoid the fourth dimension. I rarely call anyone a victim, as I believe that most people have their destiny in their own hands. But I make an exception in the case of cancer patients who are victimised by fear from the medical system.

Are they stuck in the fourth dimension forever? Not necessarily. Many unfortunate souls have been liberated from that nonluminous place by the prayers and meditations of devout people who have managed to shine light into the darkness. During deep meditation, many dedicated priests, ministers, and other prayer warriors have seen these souls coming toward them. An enlightened guru can direct spiritual people in effective spiritual work that releases ghostly ones from the shadows. They contact lost souls and tell them to go into the light, encouraging them not to be frightened. Enlightened people who are accustomed to using positive energy can actually help them with energetic thrusts. If you are interested in helping, you can find books on lost soul retrieval.

A Frenchwoman named Teresa contacted me by phone because she didn't feel quite right in spite of living a very healthy lifestyle. Though she couldn't quite put her finger on it, she was very worried that some serious condition was lurking in her system. This is a familiar story; many people call me when doctors fail to make a diagnosis and dismiss patients with "it's all in your head." It's extremely stressful to know something's wrong with you and not know what it is.

I could see that Teresa's field was entirely gray. However, after two sessions during which I strengthened her bone marrow and her liver, I told her I could not work with her. At this stage in the healing, I expected her field to be filled with bright colours, but it was still so dark I thought she must have been lying to me about being an addict or alcoholic. I'd asked her several times, but she'd denied it.

Teresa called back a few weeks later to ask whether an electrical shock might have caused the problem. I had asked whether she'd suffered any shocks, but she'd misinterpreted my questions, thinking I was talking about emotional shock. She'd forgotten to mention that she had suffered a severe electrical shock at her home a few years earlier. That explained the lengthy fusion I was seeing in her field. As I've explained, mobile phones cause small dark fusions in a person's field; the fusions from electric shock are elongated. She'd also had electrolysis treatments recently and remembered being very affected by walking under power lines. She even felt crawling sensations "like an army of ants" marching over her in the vicinity of electrical equipment.

Of course an electrical shock would have darkened her field, essentially putting out her lights. I was relieved to know that she'd never lied to me. Knowing why her field was jammed up, I was able to resume working with her, revving up her heart generator and sending her a tremendous amount of love energy to help her overcome the huge dose of negativity that had been implanted in her field so suddenly. Fortunately, she was able to find places in her environment that were reasonably free of negative energy and she even turned off the power to her house for hours at a time, which helped her considerably. She also maintained a stringent health regimen with regular exercise and an excellent diet. Before long, her field became clear and bright again. She's free from the fourth dimension and is working to experience the fifth. Importantly, she understands it's her lifetime objective to stay away from negative influences. After that case, I could easily identify fusion caused by electric shock in clients' energy fields.

The negativity of the fourth dimension is three times more powerful than positive energy. As it builds negative power, it eventually explodes, potentially causing huge damage and heartache. Nothing good can come from it. It's totally destructive in all ways. I work constantly trying to keep out of the fourth dimension. There is no doubt that the evil emitted from this dimension is now more powerful than ever, simply because the population is larger and there are many more negative frequencies from the array of high-tech products everyone thinks they must have. No matter how hard you work to stay positive, you still feel the weight of those frequencies.

Positive frequencies weigh only one-fourth as much as negative frequencies. Float two people in a pool, the negative one would have trouble staying afloat. I find this extraordinarily interesting. Negativity is the trigger for illness. The body actually becomes heavy, with many persons' backs breaking down trying to carry the load.

Fifth Dimension

This is the realm of unconditional love. When you touch into this dimension, the light becomes brighter and your emotions awaken as your heart generator becomes stronger. Goodness becomes palpable.

Spirituality is one of the main facets of this beautiful dimension; spiritual awareness opens here. You feel heart-centred, openhearted and connected to those you love. Family love is experienced in its highest manifestation and relationships can be repaired here.

It's easy to recognise this dimension, as love is its main facet. Here you fine tune into Divine loving energy. Any love you might have felt previously takes effect on this level as unconditional love develops. Within these heart-centred frequencies you work to bring every feeling and thought into the realm of pure love. Here I was able to completely surrender to God as resistance melted away.

I've regularly accessed the fifth dimension for years. I first found myself elevated into this lovely zone before I became a healer, going through a powerful boost experience. When I first reached the fifth dimension many years ago back in Australia, I began to have the most wonderful sixth-sense experiences. I discovered that I could read a person by using a flower, which I wrote about in *Conversations with the Body*. This was tremendously exciting for me. It was in this dimension that I met my spirit guide Racob who was so helpful with my children when they were small, years before my healing journey began. I was in the fifth dimension when I saw the translucent brightness of the Divine light in my apartment, travelled through the end of the rainbow, and I saw myself sitting on the crescent moon as though it were a rocking chair. A blue pearl came into my meditations as I established myself in a state of higher consciousness. Even my eating habits changed. For years now my diet has been very light and almost entirely organic.

Sixth Dimension

I first reached this dimension when visualising the clock on the Hawaiian beach. When both hands reached the number 12, I left the fifth dimension. The quality of love here seemed somewhat more comprehensive, as if I were in love not just with people but also with more abstract things like principles of truth and beauty. The feeling of purity was very strong here, and I felt very clearly that there was no room for error in my work. I had always been conscientious, but at this level doing everything correctly became more important than ever, whether or not it was part of my healing work. Doing everything correctly seemed easy here, not only in bodies but also in life.

Again, my heart generator connected with Divine love, creating amazing feelings of strength and depth. This affected my energy ray, which is literally guided by the power of Divine love. I became more adept at using it and could split it to work simultaneously on pairs of body parts such as eyes, bronchioles, lungs and kidneys.

I become aware that I'm working on myself every second to be pure and positive. The sixth dimension is where the quest for perfection seems possible. Walking the talk of perfection in my life really awakens here. How can I expect bodies to heal to perfection emotionally and physically if I don't set the standard in my own being?

Seventh Dimension

Entering this zone fills my heart with a sense of forgiveness. I feel spiritually strengthened by it, able to discern what really matters. I become accepting of how things are, realising from the depths of my soul what matters and what doesn't. Spiritual living reaches a state of perfection here. Your heart is so full of love for everything that's positive, the battle to eradicate negative interference becomes easier.

In this zone, it becomes clear that no one owns anything. Material things become meaningless. And yet, those who cling to material things are easy to forgive. I understand that they don't know better.

Eighth Dimension

I noticed in this dimension that my concern for the state of mankind and our planet was becoming very strong. My energy seems to steer itself toward helping all of humankind. I have wondered over the course of my journey whether my positive energy was being used to counteract destructive negativity in various parts of the world.

The power of the positive energy in the eighth dimension is so strong that such things seem possible. I've heard of people who believed that their prayers caused hurricanes to veer offshore where they hurt no one. These seemed like outlandish claims until I experienced the powerful energy of the eighth dimension.

From this level, I feel I might be an effective participant in major spiritual warfare, the battle between good and evil, God and Satan. I've read that adepts in eighth dimension energy can help calm turbulent situations all over the planet.

Can powerful positive energy diminish earthquakes, hurricanes and other natural phenomena that might otherwise produce drastic damage and large numbers of casualties? How about influencing groups of people like terrorists? Can they be rendered harmless by balancing out their negative energy with overwhelming blasts of positive high-frequency energy? Can we hold intentions to create peace and joy in the body politic in the same way that I help create health in individual bodies? It all seems reasonable to me.

The feeling of the powerful love and compassion you experience in the eighth dimension links you to immense power. We need to learn whether — and how — we can use it to help make things right for our planet.

Ninth Dimension

This is as far as I've come so far. My work is super powerful now. I'm travelling to incredible depths in the body parts and incredible heights in my spiritual explorations. The light fuses here into perfection, it stabilises to the point of no particles, therefore there is no interference with my work. This is where Einstein got stuck. At this time, I believe I've found my way through about two-thirds of the ninth dimension. But I believe there are many more dimensions to explore.

Human Power

We don't realise the strength of human power. Collective positive energy can be utilised to bring about positive changes for the Earth and all its people. For example, children, whose hearts are so pure, could jump up and down together during rest periods at schools shouting "peace, peace, peace." The kids would love it and powerful positive vibrations would be created that would move out into the world.

Chapter Thirteen
My ER

I was surprised and alarmed when an urgent phone call came at two o'clock in the morning from Millie, a 40-year-old client from London. "Robyn, as you know I'm six months pregnant now, and I had a car accident today. I rear-ended another vehicle. Could you look at me please? I'm starting to ache all over, my neck hurts, and worst of all, I'm spotting blood. I'm afraid I'll go into early labour." Her voice was shaking.

I had worked with Millie when she needed help becoming pregnant with her first child. She hadn't wanted In Vitro Fertilisation, preferring to become pregnant naturally. Apart from misalignment in her reproductive area, which had caused her extreme discomfort during menstruation, Millie was in good health and still had some healthy eggs. As it turned out, the problem lay with her husband, George. Testing revealed a low sperm count, so I worked with him for a short time as well. Ten months later, Millie and George got pregnant, much to the joy and delight of family and friends.

And now in the middle of the night, here was Millie telling me that she was afraid that the painful whiplash injury she had suffered would hurt her baby too. I straightened her vertebrae and cleaned out the inflammation that was beginning to build. Baby was certainly upset. Apparently the seatbelt had tightened and caused it to feel exceptional pressure. I worked through baby and Millie's entire lower abdomen, making sure that the tissues were at ease and happy again. I was glad she had contacted me, as left unattended, she and her baby might have had serious complications. I am happy to say that Millie had no adverse effects from her injuries, the pregnancy went full term, and the baby was born in perfect condition.

I have to override my own fear to take on emergency-room cases when time is of the essence. More than anything, I want to help traumatised bodies but must admit it sometimes seems overwhelming, as I've no formal emergency training. I'm a very sensitive person and feel fear that is more like responsibility, just as the next person does. I must admit that at times it can become overwhelming, but no matter how I might feel, I am extremely careful to work quickly and precisely to help these bodies in trouble.

Some ER clients call at odd hours because they're in pain from pressure in their heads or because of global time differences. If I've performed neurological work, inflammation may build up. The pressure can be extremely uncomfortable for a while until the inflammation drains away. I would rather they call me than take a painkiller. I've become very fast at removing and draining inflammation even when I'm half asleep.

I awoke one morning to a terrifying fax from Rick, a prominent magistrate in the UK, stating that his wife, Louisa, had been kicked in the liver by one of their horses and was in intensive care. Rick and Louisa had become more like friends than clients as I'd done much work with Louisa to free her from a number of ailments and had become fond of her and her husband.

She'd originally come to me having been diagnosed with a deep vein thrombosis (DVT) in her leg years earlier. She reported suffering great discomfort as the clot left her leg and moved higher into her groin. It also created other problems with digestion, circulation and an immune system that had become so weak, she caught every virus going around. She also had spells of breathlessness that her doctors, with all of their tests, could not explain.

Louisa's case of DVT was severe. This lovely young woman had not been able to stand up for more than 30 seconds, as her blood had difficulty in getting back to the heart through the damaged vein. She wore thick surgical stockings all day and used an electric pump attached to a sleeve surrounding her leg that inflated and deflated to push her blood back up toward the heart. In spite of her condition, she had borne three children in a period of six years. She'd tried "every type of healing," had seen many specialists and was having weekly session of physiotherapy. Her physical therapist had heard about me and suggested that she give me a call.

Louisa first contacted me at the end of February 2004 and started her sessions soon thereafter. She told me only about her leg, but when I did my first scan, I could see the other problems she suffered from. I also saw that her breathing problem stemmed from lungs that had never fully developed. After four sessions, I could not understand why her leg was still so painful. Only then did she mention that she was using an electric pump on it. I asked her to stop immediately, as the electrical current it was sending through her body was doing more harm than good. I also asked her to take off her surgical stockings and throw them away. Bless her heart, Louisa had become so dependent upon these gadgets, she was reluctant to put them aside. But she did, and within a few sessions, her leg began to mend.

I suggested soaking in Epsom salts and vinegar baths any time her leg began to hurt to help dispel toxicity that tended to gather there.

Before long, Louisa's health began to improve and she was happy to be able to shop, cook, play with her children, and take part in other everyday activities the rest of us take for granted. The quality of her life improved many times over. I always loved working with her, as she was conscientious about doing all of the things I suggested she do. She showed horses, so we had another bond.

And then came this foreboding fax from Rick, that I awoke to one morning. The fax said that Louisa had been kicked by a horse, and had suffered near-mortal injuries, and was not expected to pull through.

At 11:15 am I received the telephone call that we had arranged. Rick told me that Louisa had been kicked in the lower chest/abdomen by a horse and an ambulance had been called. In the hospital approximately one hour later, the accident and emergency department told me that she was too unstable to be scanned medically, because her blood pressure was fluctuating wildly. A CT scan revealed very severe lacerations to her liver, although the liver had not ruptured. They decided to leave off operating and keep her under observation at the High Dependency Unit/Intensive Care (HDU) where she could be carefully monitored in case the liver ruptured. In that case they could operate immediately. They said that the next 48-72 hours were critical. When her husband asked if she would survive they said they did not know.

Rick was in shock about the accident and dismayed that hospital personnel had said it was possible that her "liver might erupt."

"What is their plan?" I asked.

"No plan. They'll wait and see," he answered.

Although shaken, I had to act, I wasn't going to wait and see. My mind raced. I don't like working in a hospital situation because of the huge amount of electronic equipment there. But I had to do something immediately to keep her liver from rupturing. Taking a deep breath, I mentally replayed part of a conversation from a phone call Louisa had made to me weeks before.

Fortunately, I am able to replay the sound of people's voices from previous encounters or telephone conversations even if it had been only a few words. From that I am able to tune into their vibration, which gives me access to their bodies. In fact, I am able to make a connection if a person simply tells me about someone close to them who is not feeling well. For example, if a wife tells me about her husband, I am able to make a diagnosis for him through speaking with his wife.

I tuned into the vibration of Louisa's voice and then went straight to her liver. It was in tremendous shock. I located the lesions on her liver, and then surrounded the suffering organ with love, just as though I had my arms around it. I said to it: "You will be okay, we'll get you well."

I stayed with Louisa day and night, working around the clock for 48 hours, acting as a life support machine. The only way I can describe it is to say that I worked in a cycle: liver, lungs, and heart, working even during my light evening naps. I would awaken knowing I hadn't ceased and was still cycling through the troubled areas. Finally, it became clear to me that Louisa would live. Knowing this, I gave way to total exhaustion for a short time. Of course there would be more to do to restore her liver, but the crisis was over and I took time to renew my own strength before working with Louisa on the phone.

First Day

Rick saw to it that Louisa had a landline phone at her bedside. On our first actual phone session on March 23, 2005, she was in deep shock, not very coherent. She was on a saline drip and was being administered morphine. I encouraged them to use a gentler painkiller, as a numbed body is very difficult to heal; it forgets to kick into natural healing mode. Louisa was on the list for emergency surgery. The liver, gallbladder and lungs were not functioning to produce clean, quality blood, and her heart was beginning to fail. It was also in severe shock. The right side of her lung was bruised and her shoulder was also damaged. A neck vertebra, C3, was out of alignment.

Second Day

My work had contained the liver from rupture and so the next day, I worked on strengthening all the other areas that were damaged. Louisa did not sound strong. I concentrated on stretching the bile duct to help the liver to function. Also the heart arteries needed help. The timing of valves had to be reset and fluid and blood had to be removed from the lungs. I then made an exit at the base of the lungs so infection could drain away.

Third Day

Louisa was still in serious trouble, her heart rate was down to 32 beats per minute and she had an extremely high temperature. Over the next 48 hours, I literally become Louisa's life support machine to keep the liver, gallbladder, lungs and heart functioning. Further stretching of the arteries was done and I continued working on all the body and cleaning the energy field of negative interference. It is very difficult to keep the field clean in hospitals because they are full of electronic instruments, to say nothing of the low frequency levels from so many people in trouble. It was almost impossible to stay ahead of all of these negative influences.

Fourth Day

Louisa had picked up an infection, which entered through the catheter into the bladder. Her system was trying desperately to keep it out of the liver. I did what I could to help

Fifth Day

Louisa was still in severe pain from the deep bruising. I could see that a mass had collected outside the right lung area, which was inflamed, infected and contained thickened blood. It had also been picked up on the hospital scan. I worked to remove it.

Rick was now desperate as well and shock was badly affecting him. I worked on him enough to keep him functioning. I was concerned that Louisa had become weak from lack of nourishment, as the hospital had not given any through the drip. I gave Richard instructions for preparing nourishing broth. Over the next weeks, I was to give him enough recipes to fill a cookbook.

Sixth Day

Louisa was starting to pick up. Rick was very upset with the quality of care at the hospital and moved her to a private hospital. Louisa's body now had to attempt to cope with a type of poisoning from the saline drip being left in too long.

Seventh Day

The care in the second hospital was much better. Louisa could now stand up for brief times. I continued to work on her daily.

Louisa was released from the hospital Friday, April 8, two weeks after the accident. By early May, she was again enjoying robust health.

Working as a life support machine was exhausting, to say the least. Even in my light sleep periods, I was aware of constantly working with her liver, lungs and heart. Both Rick and Louisa sent me glowing letters of thanks after she was happy and healthy at home once again. Hers was a healing I will never forget.

• • • •

At 5 a.m. one Thursday morning, I was flying through various brilliant levels of colour with friends when the ringing of my bedside phone shattered my magnificent dream.

The woman on the phone was crying, "Robyn, I'm not sure of the time difference, I just wanted to hear your voice. My pain is excruciating. It's my spinal nerves again."

"Okay, Janet, give me ten minutes to wake up and I'll see what I can do."

Janet and I had been working on her back and the rest of her body for a while. She was perhaps the most evolved person I had ever worked with, a wonderful soul, and I was happy to hear from her again.

When she had first found me, she told me the story of how she'd slipped and fallen down a flight of stairs forty years previously, bouncing down step after step on her coccyx. Since her fall, Janet had seen doctors, physical therapists, chiropractors, osteopaths, acupuncturists and everyone else she could think of, but her pain kept getting worse. Painkilling drugs did not relieve the acute pain and she was opposed to drugs on principle. She'd become dispirited and her general health suffered with various infections. Several months before she first contacted me, she'd had magnetic resonance imaging (MRI) from which her surgeon diagnosed "nerve root entrapment of the spine and a marked degree of spinal canal narrowing." He felt surgery was too risky and the radiologist concurred adding that no medication would alleviate the pain and no treatment would help her condition.

Janet hadn't known how she could continue to walk, even with her walking stick, as her right side had become considerably shorter than her left. She had been afraid there was nothing left for her but life in a wheelchair, a dreadful prospect for a woman who loved her formerly active life. During our first session, she had mentioned often being in tears with excruciating pain. "Negative feelings have taken over," she said and I heard deep sadness in her voice.

During our first session, I found a sugar imbalance, poor circulation and weakness of the pituitary gland and heart valves. She was "stunned" when I mentioned that a hepatitis virus had affected her liver 18 years previously. She then remembered that she'd contracted Myalgic Encephalopathy (ME) at that time after a holiday abroad. I also repaired a 20-year-old head injury she had completely forgotten. Her hips were also painful. In the lower back I found shriveled nerves on the right side, which I was sure was what her doctor referred to as "nerve root entrapment," the source of her pain. I worked to straighten and strengthen the nerve fibers.

On subsequent sessions, I checked and strengthened

her body, doing all I could to relieve her pain by cleaning inflammation from the nerves of the spine. This would be the crucial part for the success of her healing. Little did I realise when we started that Janet's case would become one of my most exciting.

And now on this early morning, she called back and we went forward into more unusual healing. I hoped it was time for the next part of our work, to stretch her right side three inches to realign her spine and leg. I had realigned bodies previously, but three inches was going to be a huge challenge, even though I believed I could do it. But first I had to scan her body to get it ready. My scan revealed her spine from C-1 down to L-2 was super strong and straight from our previous work. I did all I could to relieve her pain by cleaning the nerves of inflammation from the L-2 vertebra through to her tailbone. There was still calcification around her right hip, pelvic bone and her coccyx, which I had to clean prior to our stretching exercises.

I asked Janet to lie flat on the floor on her back. Then I asked her to point her toes to the ceiling and lengthen her right leg. While she held the length she had obtained, I worked from her hip through the pelvic area and the leg itself to hold the length we had made. I visualise her skeleton at the end of each realignment session, facing her structure from behind. I then dangle it. It's usually wobbly. My objective is to hold it straight, which takes huge strength and focus on my part.

I also gave Janet reaching exercises to perform with her arms between sessions. Gradually we obtained the desired realignment.

Janet's healing was speeded by her enthusiasm for doing the exercises and taking the supplements I'd recommended. She also listened to my PMP messages, which she says helped her considerably.

Spinal injuries take time to heal but before long, her mood and health improved to the extent that friends complimented her on how well she looked and her husband was amazed at the changes taking place. She wrote me a lovely thank-you note telling me that she'd regained her energy and self-confidence. Even her eyesight had improved, causing her to seek new lenses from her optician. She told me how she loves to look at herself in passing shop windows to view how straight she is now. She has no more fear of crutches or wheelchairs.

• • • •

It's one thing to handle emergency situations involving well-established clients I know and care for, quite another to administer care to a total stranger. During a flight to Australia on an Asian airline, I was in the restroom when an announcement came over the loudspeaker: "Is there a doctor on board?" I wondered what the problem was as I washed my hands. Then again, "Is there a doctor on board?" The stewardess's voice sounded distressed now. No Robyn, don't even think about it, I told myself.

Then again the announcement came, this time sounding very agitated. I took a deep breath and opened the door to find three stewardesses standing right there as though they were waiting for me.

"I'm a natural practitioner, I'll do what I can," I said.

"It's a young girl," one of them replied, "she is unconscious, come with us, she's down the front." By now the panic-stricken mother had joined us. Actually they were all panic-stricken.

We quickly trotted up the aisle and by the time we were ten seats away, I could see her slumped in her seat. "Her blood pressure is down," I stated.

"How you know that?" asked the mother in her Asian English.

"Er, oh, medical people know these things," I boldly answered. By this time we had reached the girl, a young teenager.

As no doctor had come forth, I knew it was up to me. The mother's panic was very upsetting and I realised that in order to make her comfortable with my efforts, I'd have to look "professional." Placing my hand on the girl's forehead just as a physician would do, I went into my zone. It's her heart, I thought. Next I picked up her wrist to take her pulse. I was working desperately inside the girl and had no need to take her pulse, but her mother would find comfort in seeing familiar gestures. Within a few minutes, the girl started to come to. Of course, the mother was ecstatic.

"Are you okay?" I asked the girl, who by now had some colour returning to her face.

"Yes I feel really good," she answered.

I left the mother with instructions to take the girl to her regular physician as soon as the plane landed to have her checked out. I knew she was all right, but wanted to make sure the mother would not go on worrying.

The stewardesses and the mother bowed with their hands together in front of them. So charming. "Thank you, thank you," they were saying.

I checked on the girl later in the flight, she was doing very well indeed. She and her mother will never really know how her life was saved at 35,000 feet above the ocean.

Chapter Fourteen
Into a Healthy Twenty-First Century

I find it ironic that the hardworking "Greatest Generation" followed a healthy lifestyle while many modern people, who have so much more material wealth, live lives filled with unhealthy stress. Today we're much more likely to rely on drugs to cure disease than on commonsense living that prevents it in the first place.

My first memory of healthcare came from my beloved maternal grandmother, Granny Penny. We visited her every Sunday for a big dinner and I can remember these occasions vividly.

Granny would greet us wearing a big smile and an immaculate frilly apron over her Sunday dress. The family gathered from here and there, my aunts and cousins and everyone else. Granny managed to keep up with every conversation while tending to the delicious dishes she was cooking on her Aga cooker. No doubt I learned from her the fun of entertaining and cooking for people.

The mantle above the cooker where she stored small utensils had scalloped fabric hanging from its edge. The smooth stone floor was covered with colourful crocheted cotton fabric mats. A long wooden table covered with one of Granny's white crocheted tablecloths stood proudly in the centre of the room. My grandmother was renowned for her handcrafts — I always loved watching patterns emerging as she created lovely articles with her aged hands.

Some Sundays prior to lunch, my cousins and I would be called for our dose of castor oil. Even on the drive there I would be asking my parents "It's not castor oil day is it?" My cousins seemed to take it in stride, but I would start dry retching waiting my turn. Maybe my taste buds were more sensitive than my cousins' were.

Granny Penny set the standard for my parents, who made sure that every other day of the week we had cod liver oil, milk of magnesia and vitamin C. And today we know this old wives tail of feeding kids cod liver oil has been proven by research to result in measurably more intelligent children. Give any children in your care 2000 mg of fish oil daily.

And take 4000 mg yourself daily. And let them have butter if they're hungry for it. Their developing brains are probably looking for the fat called arachidonic acid present in butter. But no, never margarine. We were also wormed annually. Our food was grown naturally and we had Chinese vegetable gardens behind our land. Our eggs were always fresh as my father kept a chook run, the Australian term for a chicken coup or house.

Many of my clients remember similar childhood scenes but sadly, much of the sensible healthcare of that generation disappeared when fashionable pills and chemical drugs arrived on the scene. Manufacturers took over. But now, thank heavens, many people are returning to natural commonsense ways of Granny Penny's era. Experts are now suggesting family gatherings, where delicious meals are served, to bolster body, mind and spirit. Many of us know we should purchase organic produce and try to find spring water, even if we have to pay for bottles shipped in from other locations.

Drinking Water

I took a break from my busy schedule in Vancouver to visit my friends in Seattle. We attended a spellbinding lecture by Dr Masaru Emoto, the celebrated natural healing doctor and author of several books including *The Hidden Messages In Water* that have sold millions of copies worldwide. His research on the responsive, emotional qualities of water crystals is amazing and his photographs of drops of water are worth a trip to your bookstore or library to see. I was pleased to hear him say that Vancouver is the only Western city he has tested that has pure tap water.

His work underscores what we've been told for ages: Because the human body is 85 percent fluid, it's very important to drink pure water and plenty of it. Scientists are now finding evidence that atoms and molecules in water have a spin and can in some instances spin anticlockwise, which is against the natural flow of energy. I've observed that healthy cells spin to the right but if a person has a disease like cancer, their cells will be spinning counterclockwise

This means that water spinning to the right is scattering energy, as in an explosion. Turning to the left is toward the direction of implosion, which increases energy. The healing water of Lourdes, France has been found to have a left spin, meaning strong energy. This energy is transferred to the person drinking it.

Some investigators believe that 95 percent of drinking water, no matter where it comes from, is spinning the unhealthy way. In London, people joked about tap water being purified urine, having been filtered through thirteen sets of kidneys — but it's no joke to people who have painful kidney stones.

Vegetables and Fruits

Are organic foods worth the extra cost? I have to give that a qualified yes, although even in that supposedly spotless industry, some growers, shippers, and vendors unscrupulously label things organic that really are not. A reliable grocer is your best protection, one that's been in business for a while and who is trustworthy.

Vegetables can also be a source of parasitic contamination. If you buy your vegetables in prepackaged plastic, salads in bags, for example, make sure you wash them thoroughly no matter what the package promises. While some are washed before packaging, don't take a chance that they've been washed enough. You can soak lettuce and other veggies in water with a few ounces of white vinegar added to kill germs and remove at least some of the pesticides.

Tropical fruit is among the healthiest foods now. Much of it is still grown naturally and suits our bodies at this stage of our development. I have noted that many who thought vegetarianism was the way to go are now quite sensibly including animal protein in their diets again. We're not ready to become vegetarians, though we're heading in that direction. I believe it will take another two lifetimes.

Meat and Poultry

We no longer require red meat unless we are doing heavy work. I still need it sometimes if I have been working out more energetically than usual. Poultry is a good choice, especially if you can find fowl that has not been fed antibiotics and hormones. Legs and thighs contain the most nutrition and energy. As carnivores, we need protein six of seven days a week in an amount equivalent to the size of your clenched fist.

I suggest that you wash off every piece of meat and

poultry before cooking, especially if you bought it already wrapped in plastic, which makes good bacteria breeding ground. As with everything else, the source of your meat is important. Ideally you could drive out to an organic ranch and have your meat butchered for you, but very few people are in a position to do so. We have to rely on our grocery stores and butcher shops to sell us safe meat. Wash your hands with strong soap after handling raw poultry and meat. You can also purchase boxes of inexpensive disposable plastic gloves to use in your kitchen.

Fish

Wholesome wild fish are the perfect protein food now, but you have to be very careful that your source of supply is 100 percent reliable. I have already mentioned dangers of farmed seafood. "Global" merchants are wreaking havoc on our fish supply, importing and exporting species to new breeding grounds and along with them, diseases and parasites from their original locations that wipe out wild fish. I'm not saying that all fish farming companies are selling us contaminated fish. Not by any means. But there are enough who do to make the others come under suspicion as well. Atlantic salmon is now being "farmed" in the Pacific Ocean off the coast of Chile. Most of these farms are reasonably sanitary but a few are disgustingly dirty and local fishermen who depend on wild fish for a living are lodging complaints. (And in addition, the farmed fish do not contain the precious Omega 3 fish oils since these fish are fed grain, not krill and plankton.)

Asian fish are being introduced to the waters off Mexico, where native species have no defenses against the notoriously devastating Asian tapeworms and other parasites and bacteria they bring with them. If at all possible, avoid farmed fish. Yes, it is cheaper, but not if it makes you sick — and it will if you take one look at the crowded unsanitary pens where many poor fish are "raised." How can miserable diseased fish nourish humans? Australia is the only country that by law has to state on the price tag that it's imported. You might want to send a note to your government representative asking for such protection in your country.

Obesity

Obesity is now a major problem. Sugar is the major culprit. It's found in almost everything now in the form of corn syrup, even some packages of frozen vegetables. Be sure you read labels carefully and avoid it at all costs.

The other major culprit are the starchy foods. Look at starch and sugar as 'fuel' foods. You know that starch is composed of long chains of sugar molecules, strung together like a string of beads. Digestion is what breaks this string apart, releasing the individual sugar molecules.

Then in the cell, sugar along with oxygen is what our cells use to combust and produce energy. However if we consume more fuel foods than we are burning, our bodies will most surely save this extra fuel. To save it, the liver, under the direction of insulin, takes 3 molecules of sugar and converts it into one molecule of fat. This fat is called triglyceride, and could be called liquid fat. It can be measured in the cholesterol panel. This liquid fat called triglyceride will eventually be deposited in the belly as solid fat.

So the size of the belly becomes the indicator of how much extra fuel you have been consuming over the years.

We have been scared off of eating fat, being told that it is fat in the diet that makes us fat. As a result of this erroneous thinking, we have, if anything, become fat deficient, though this is a crucial food.

The best fat to consume is fish oil either as fish itself, or in the form of capsules. Next best is Olive oil — eat it in your salad, and do your light frying with it. And don't be scared off of coconut oil. It has many benefits even though it is a saturated fat. All that is meant by the term saturated fat is that the oil or fat is solid at room temperature. It is erroneously assumed that because animal fat is a saturated fat, all saturated fat must be bad for you. In the case of coconut, nothing could be further from the truth. It is not at all like the other saturated fats with which it has been identified.

So to summarise, limit your intake of fuel foods, the sugar and the starch, eat your fist-size of protein daily and be sure to get fish oil and olive oil and coconut oil daily.

We have become too busy to cook so the majority buy take-out, much of which is loaded with fat, particularly the notoriously damaging trans fats used for frying — especially for french fries. New York City recently prohibited restaurants from cooking with trans fats and other cities are implementing similar rules. But that's only part of the problem. Other fats add calories and much of take-away is high in carbohydrates as well. Obesity is leading to high incidences of diabetes. It's estimated that 40 million Americans are obese, with millions more in others countries. In my work, I instantly know that the client has a sugar imbalance when I see three of the four following organs malfunctioning: duodenals, pancreas, spleen and adrenals. Once the organs are restored to wellness the problem goes. However, my work cannot restore a body that has been receiving insulin for a length of time.

Arthritic Extremities

The force of gravity drains acid toxin into our hands and feet where it creates pain and bone damage. This is especially true if your liver has not been performing its detox functions. A bowel that is not open can have the same effect. The point of origin has to be healed, however, to help with pain you can soak your hands and feet in a bucket of warm water containing two cups of Epsom salts and one of cider vinegar. This helps toxins leave via the pores in your skin. There are more sweat glands in feet than anywhere else in the body — about 2,500 of them. Many people have told me of dark rims of toxin surrounding the tub if they've had a full bath containing four large mugs of Epsom salts and two of vinegar.

Vinegar

This amazingly versatile product is useful around the house and also offers health benefits. It has been used in remedies since Biblical times and in ancient Babylon and Rome. I advise having both white vinegar and cider vinegar on hand.

High quality cider vinegar, organic and aged in the wood, is used in many folk remedies. This lovely vinegar is a golden colour and should be a bit cloudy. The sediment is referred to as "mother of vinegar."

A teaspoon or two of cider vinegar mixed into a glass of water can be taken morning and evening to adjust the pH level of your body, the acid/alkaline balance. This may be effective in preventing urinary tract irritation, stomach ulcers, high blood pressure, high LDL cholesterol, kidney stones, gallstones, and other conditions that an overly acid system may contribute to. You can also use cider vinegar in salads, soups, sauces, and dressings to add a touch of flavour along with the health benefits it offers.

Cider vinegar is thought to be a remedy for nausea, with two teaspoonfuls stirred into a glass of water recommended four times a day. Some recommend soaking a clean cloth in warm vinegar and placing it over your stomach while lying down.

White distilled vinegar can be used to soak vegetables and fruits to take at least some of the pesticides away. Just pour a few ounces into a sink full of water and soak your produce for twenty minutes or so. You can keep undiluted white vinegar in a spray bottle to use on bathroom and kitchen counters and fixtures. It's a great deodorant for garbage cans, boats, camping equipment and anything else that gets musty. Toenail fungus which makes nails thick and yellow can be helped with a few drops of undiluted white vinegar on them morning and night. By changing the pH balance around the nails, you're radically changing the fungi's environment and they die.

Exercise

We all sit too much, and fail to get enough exercise. We sit to eat, to drive or take public transportation, and increasingly we sit all day at work — and sometimes on into the night. The human body needs to work; its energy needs to be used. I've noticed that people in the UK walk more than those in the rest of the world. Though I cannot be sure whether walking is the reason, I consistently see when I scan their bodies that their glands are larger and stronger than those of people in other countries are. Exercise is becoming more popular in other parts of the world, thank goodness, especially on the West Coast of America, in Vancouver and Australia. Still there are too many Americans who'll automatically hop in their cars to drive two blocks. Pity, as their bodies need to be revved up far more than their engines do and they are creating pollution. I have not owned a car for 15 years.

Aging and lack of exercise bring on body structure weakness. While we cannot do anything about aging, we can do quite a lot to keep the effects at a minimum. I agree with the experts who now recommend an hour of vigorous exercise 4-5 days a week to keep the heart healthy and the skeleton strong. Bad posture is the cause of many back problems. It tends to get worse over the years. Sitting slumped or sitting on the back of the buttocks rather than the front places more pressure on the tailbone and sciatic nerves. So stand and sit tall.

Carrying the load of life as it is today is immense. Spines are in terrible trouble, much weaker than they were sixty odd years ago. Between lack of exercise and the weakening effects of chemical and radiation pollution, any damage from accidents is very difficult to overcome.

John, a sixty-three-year-old American, called asking for help with back pain. He described "intense pain in my lower back, tail bone area and neck area of the spine. These pains are the results of three injuries over the past thirty or so years. My work at the time required moderate to heavy lifting for extended periods of time on a regular basis.

I came to this job with two vertebras that were injured in 1973, resulting in a crack in each one. About eight months ago, I slipped and hit my tailbone on a sharp corner of a cabinet, causing excruciating pain for a number of weeks and required me to use a pillow whenever I sat to drive."

After our first two sessions, John was amazed. "My tailbone pains were completely eradicated, and have not since returned." It took a longer time to get his entire spine into solid alignment, but before long, John was satisfied with the results and could again work as hard as his job required.

John is one of millions of working people whose jobs depend upon the health of their spines. If their backs give out, they lose their source of income. It distresses me to know that so many people walk around in excruciating pain. Here's an easy exercise that should be helpful for many if not all back pain sufferers.

Dangle Back Exercise

This exercise aids the separation of discs and vertebrae and helps to clear inflammation. It is very important to do it first thing in the morning. You can perform it up to five more times throughout the day.

Spread your feet about twelve inches apart. Moving very gently, bend forward and allow your hands and arms to hang heavy toward the floor. Hold this dangling position until the first sign of discomfort.

Slowly straighten up. Stand still and breathe the Breath of Life twice, affirming "perfect back, perfect back."

Again, gently bend forward and dangle. You may notice that each time you dangle, your fingertips get a little closer to the floor.

Don't ever ask too much of your back during this exercise. The moment it complains, gently straighten up. Persevere. Improvement comes slowly but it will happen.

Unnecessary Back Surgery

Thankfully, I was able to help Sany, a young woman who had undergone needless back surgery. She had suffered pain in her back and legs since the birth of her child and was eventually diagnosed with Cauda Equina Syndrome, a rare disorder affecting the bundle of nerve roots at the lower (lumbar) end of the spinal cord. Her doctor told her that a slipped disc in her lumbar region was affecting the nerve leading to the bladder, creating problems. To prevent further permanent damage to the nerve, she would need "disc decompression" surgery. Not knowing what else she might do, she acquiesced.

I heard from Sany as she was convalescing. After a few sessions she felt better but I was not satisfied with our progress. Then I saw a strange silver glow just to the left of her operation site. It looked something like metal surgical clips I'd seen in several post-op clients in the past, but I was not quite sure that's what I was seeing here. I worked to remove scar tissue to get a better look. During our next session, I was able to discern that the silver glow had a distinct curved shape. It was not a clip. She then realised I was seeing her contraceptive coil, which had been there for a number of years and was now badly out of place.

"Sany, have it taken out immediately," I advised. Following my recommendation, she went to her doctor's clinic where they removed it. She told me that immediately afterward she felt "a lightness within my body." She also reported beneficial changes in her spine during our next sessions. There is no doubt in my mind that had the coil been removed first, Sany's spinal surgery would have been unnecessary.

If you use an Intrauterine Device (IUD) as Sany did, please have it checked annually. They're not meant to last forever and may cause infections and other problems.

The Healer's Job

As healers, I believe we must be in radiant health and disciplined in body, mind and soul. I work very hard to walk the talk. I'm always surprised when I hear of healers who are not well people. I cannot imagine how they can expect another body to become healthy and strong if they do not provide a blueprint for it in their own bodies. Positive energy has to be triple strength to combat and evade the negative intruder in the temple of the body. In one popular healing technique, "point holders," most of whom are not in good health either, surround the ailing person lying on the table. Where is the positive energy needed to make the patient well?

Healing, like most other changes, has become a whole new ballgame. We certainly won't go back to candle light. The day has gone where one was born and expected to live a long healthy life experiencing nothing but the usual change-of-weather cold. Staying well now has to be acknowledged in a far different manner, our energy fields are the human part that needs the most help. Tend your field, feed it positive energy, keep it clean of negative invasion and your body will be well, it's as simple as that.

How can you reach higher dimensions where healing takes place? A calm, steady mind is the key. The mind stilling exercise in Chapter 12 will help you control your mind. You must be able to still your mind and concentrate your full attention on the work if you want to succeed.

Effective Natural Remedies

I'm not out to replace the medical establishment by any means but I do know of some wonderful natural remedies that are fairly inexpensive and worth a try. I have found a wonderful natural antibiotic that seems to work as advertised. It's called olive leaf oil extract, made from the olive tree. I'm very impressed. In my experience, it's on a par with vitamin E for healing open wounds and does a wonderful job for infections.

Everyone should give his or her liver an annual birthday present of a bottle of milk thistle. I still see the need for this herb to help your liver, as in an increasingly polluted world, its work now is immense. No matter how careful you are, preservatives are still a huge concern as they add to body sluggishness and jam the liver. I suggest you eliminate canned goods from your kitchen shelves and anything else containing artificial preservatives, as they cause digestive upset.

I have found nothing to replace good old castor oil, as it gets into nooks and crannies like no other substance. You can also train your bowel to respond to your urging. Just say to it, "Okay bowel we need a clean out," and if you're persistent, you bowel will learn to respond after just a bit of coaxing. I do recommend an annual dose of castor oil to make sure. And yes, I take it myself.

Epsom salt and vinegar baths are still the best detoxifiers. Pour four large coffee mugs of Epsom salts and two of cider vinegar into a deep warm tub and soak for twenty minutes. On the first week have three long soaks, two the following week, and then once a week from then on.

As I've said, my healing techniques advance over time. In a similar way, medical care is advancing as well. One of the techniques that has saved patients hours of painful recovery time is keyhole or arthroscopic surgery, which eliminates the need for such large incisions to get the job done.

Having seen the devastating results from body parts being carelessly tucked back into body cavities after surgery, I'm especially pleased to know that these poor little organs will no longer be puzzled about where they belong. Every part of the human body has its home, its own living space. And they so much enjoy the "comforts of home", and being in company with their dear friends.

Colons seem to be the organs most carelessly handled. I have seen too many ascending and descending colons unable to function correctly because of displacement. I find this heartbreaking and disrespectful. I would like physicians to be kinder toward body parts and to stop using so many chemical poisons to heal the body.

How effective are these drugs anyway? A recent report stated that for every $1 spent on medication, consumers spend an additional $1.50 to purchase pills to counteract side effects. I find that nothing short of mind boggling. I can unequivocally state from my findings that the body can and does heal without medication or with very low dosage. I've proved it time and time again.

Conversations with the Body

As I wrote in my recent book, *Conversations with the Body*, loving the body is very important. When I go inside a body and see and feel the suffering of body parts, I do all I can to restore and help them fulfill their destiny. All they want is to do their work as they have been programmed to do by our Creator. When you lie down at night, think about the body temple you live in, and send warm loving energy to every part of it. Talk to it, thank it for getting you through another day, let it know that you care.

Then, focus on any problem area you may have. Picture the problem clearing up as you surround the affected part with your strong emotion of love. This can help with any part of your body, especially if you can work this method while you're in high vibration levels. My *Dimensional Healing* CD is a great help as it takes you there.

Conversing with your body like this may seem strange to you at first, but if you keep it up for a number of nights it will soon become a habit. After a while, you will get answers from your organs in the form of small flutters that say 'I hear you.' I believe that if you do not love a body part, it may feel inadequate and decide to leave. For example 90 percent of my clients with breast cancer had openly talked of not being happy with either the size or shape of their breasts. Such negativity and vanity almost insult the true purpose of the breasts and can create another body weakness.

Pleasure is also important. Your body needs to be rewarded for the fine work it does. Here are some suggestions for making life pleasant for various parts of your body:

Eyes: Look for beauty, seek and find love, feed it through the eyes to the heart generator.

Nose: Inhale lovely fragrances, especially when doing your deep, positive reprogramming breath exercise. Positive smells beautiful, negative smells bad.

Ears: Be a good listener. Hear the sounds of birds, nature and melodious, harmonic music.

Mouth: Taste. Enhance your taste buds. Listen to what your mouth tells you. As you climb into higher levels of awareness, your taste buds will warn you of chemicals in an area; the back of your mouth will taste metallic. When that happens, leave the area as soon as possible. I find that shops selling building supplies and household contents affect me.

Hands: Touch. Feel. Stroke different textures. Hug others, if they will allow you to. Caress animals. Make contact between all parts of your body and the natural world.

Feet: Walk barefoot in sand, which has huge energy because it is always moving, and also on grassy areas. Sit on the ground with your back against a tree to obtain extra energy.

All body parts: Talk to all of them with love and compassion, especially if they are sick. Reward them as they become well, telling them how clever they are.

If you have a sick kidney, for example, visualise what it looks like and its location in the body. Explain to it that you know it is not well. Surround it mentally with love and ask it to help you get rid of negative influences affecting it. Believe me, it will appreciate the team support you are giving it and will no longer feel alone while battling for regained health.

Your love helps your body to ward off invasion of negative energy, germs and other forms of attack. This sort of communication establishes a permanent link to your body parts.

A happy, well-exercised, well-nourished body should stay strong for many, many, many years. You will benefit in countless ways from helping your body do the many things required to keep you healthy.

The Future of Healing

In the future, I see the healing done by using vibrational doses, which will not be taken internally. When such a sophisticated technique is perfected, surgery will not be necessary unless injury is caused by an accident. Today, we have the erroneous attitude: "cut it out, you don't need that body part," but we do need all of our parts for superior functioning. Would your car run well with some of its parts missing?

Evolution is speeding up, but the problem is most of us have not kept up with developments. Soon humans will be able to tap into the quantum zone, to have the ability to turn up or lower this energy source like a dimmer switch on a light globe. We will become the switch to turn on this natural power.

Having this control of power, resourceful people will produce natural technology to overcome the negativity of today's energy supply that is so damaging to our health. We have to learn to live in this technological world we have made. If you think the past fifty years have brought about huge development, just wait for the next fifty.

The really exciting possibilities lie in coming to understand energy, the way we use it, the effect it has on us and accept that it is what we are. This is the first century that we have walked under electrical wires and coped with all the products this power gives life to. These inventions came from the human because they are us. Our energy fields have light from natural power and the ability to hold positive or negative frequencies. Our fields are computerised; we are constantly taking photos, storing them in our memories, and sending and receiving messages. We are all the products we invented. Alexander Graham Bell's wife was deaf. In his endeavour to help her hear he did extensive research into the human hearing system, and came up with the telephone. The first structured design for bridges to span rivers came from the inside of bone. I'm the human version of the endoscope, but because of the rigidity of the manufactured version, it can't get around corners as I can.

Despite our inherent power, most humans tend to dismiss their souls and intelligence and give power to material products. Sometimes I think human beings are becoming like machines. In Japan, a robot was invented that looks exactly like Einstein. Where's the respect? Gone with our soul's sensitivity, I suspect.

Respect and love go hand in hand. You will never love someone you don't respect. Now our respect is dwindling for ourselves and other people because we are focusing our affection, desire, and even love on material products. The first time I asked attendees of my seminar to leave mobile phones outside the room I was amazed at their response. Judging by the looks on their faces, I might as well have asked them to leave an arm or leg in the hall. Canada has now labeled it as an addiction.

I'm not against progress. We have to evolve, but as we do, we will make some mistakes. It seems to me that the power we use is one of them, as it's going anticlockwise, in the negative direction. Natural energy runs clockwise as I've said in earlier chapters. Mother Nature is angry and unless we accept responsibility for cleaning up the mess we've made, I dare not think of the consequences.

We forget we are just stewards passing through. We need to leave the planet in good shape for future generations. As I have always said, negative energy is three times stronger than positive energy, until explosion, we have birthed a new energy, and by doing so given access to negative explosions. You would think that from all the explosions going on now that mankind would realise that something is wrong.

So many changes have taken place in the last fifty or

sixty years, it seems that our parents' generation was born into an entirely different world. Here's a list of how life looked to someone growing up in the 1950s:

We were born before television, before polio shots, frozen foods, Xerox copies, plastic, contact lenses, Frisbees and the Pill.

We were born before credit cards, split atoms, laser beams and ballpoint pens, before pantyhose, dishwashers, clothes dryers, electric blankets, air conditioners, drip-dry clothes — and before man walked on the moon.

We got married and then lived together. How quaint can you be?

In our time, closets were for clothes, not for "coming out of". Bunnies were small rabbits and rabbits were not Volkswagens. Designer Jeans were scheming girls named Jean or Jeanne, and having a meaningful relationship meant getting along well with our cousins.

We thought fast food was what you ate during Lent and outer space was the back of the Riviera Theatre.

We were born before househusbands, gay rights, computer dating, dual careers, and commuter marriages. We were born before daycare centres, group therapy and nursing homes.

We never heard of computers, FM radio, electric typewriters, artificial hearts, word processors, yogurt, and guys wearing earrings.

For us, timesharing meant togetherness, not condos or

computers; a chip was a piece of wood, hardware meant hardware and software wasn't even a word.

In 1946, "made in Japan" meant junk and the term "making out" referred to how you did on your exam. Pizzas, Macdonald's and instant coffee were unheard of.

In our day, cigarette smoking was fashionable, grass was mowed, coke was a cold drink, and pot was something you cooked in. Rock music was a grandma's lullaby and AIDS were helpers in the principal's office.

We were certainly not before the difference between the sexes was discovered but were surely before the sex change; we made do with what we had. And we were the last generation that was so dumb as to think you needed a husband to have a baby.

Interesting evolutionary changes are taking place that give me hope. In the past fifty years, evolution has been incredible. The speed has been tremendous. Many young people are repudiating materialism, instead using their energies to build a more conscious world, aware that their real purpose on earth is soul growth. Like tribal people in the past, they seek to live in harmony, taking only what was needed at the time.

The planet heartbeat used to be 7.8 cycles, it's now risen to 14.3 cycles. Even though we have angered Mother Nature she is still trying to support us, not only by giving hard lessons but also by creating changes within us to enable us to evolve. We are now experiencing a DNA change in our bodies as we go through a phase of accelerated evolution.

Some physical and mental conditions accompany the shift into more evolved life:

Sneezing

Dizziness

Occasional diarrhea

Runny nose

Body vibrating, especially at night when relaxed

Back pains

Changes in our circulation flow

Loss of limb power

Some change in breathing, stronger if anything

Lymphatic glands adjusting and readjusting

General tiredness

Oppression — for no reason

Hearts are causing concern trying to attune to our DNA change and planetary heartbeat, which is not regular now.

I know many readers will find it difficult to know the difference between signs of DNA body changes and similar symptoms from illness. I can tell you that the DNA symptoms pass when the physical work is complete. All in all we are being helped to re-attune every cell in our bodies. Fortunately, there are more evolved souls on earth today than in any other lifetime to help. Let's hope that Einstein's was right, "The philosophy of one generation is commonsense to the next."

It's so very hard to get away from the primacy of greed.

Money is behind virtually everything now. Everything is judged by its financial value. I saw very clearly where this leads on that same trip to Australia when I spent some time with an attractive man named James. He'd inherited great wealth and increased it by making excellent investments. You'd think he'd be a happy man but in reality, he was the cheapest, unhappiest human being I've ever known. His idea of making soup was to purchase half a carrot and one stick of celery at the store so as not to waste a nickel. He took joy only in watching his fortune grow. While visiting him, I sewed him a Canadian flag to replace the tattered one flying above his country property, little knowing that I'd one day live in Canada where the red maple leaf flag flies over every public building. Was that a coincidence? The big lesson I learned from my relationship with this troubled man was that material things offer little comfort in life. Collecting as much money as possible will never make anyone happy. I recently learned that this man is very ill and living with caretakers.

Something that I have definitely learned is that to be well and happy now is to approach living with an intelligent common sense attitude without paranoia. These following hints can be of use to you for the new game of wellness.

Check a ten-mile radius around your living space for electrical boxes and towers and mobile phone towers, if apparent, move.

Mend your relationships or finish them, if you forgive

do it from the bottom of your heart.

Clean your abode and body inside and out. Remove any furnishings you don't love.

Don't allow negative dumping from friends and family, in doing so try not to close doors.

Feed your body and family good healthy foods.

Feed your system loving positive thoughts.

Keep your heart area warm by feeding it love of anything, but let your conscience be your guide.

Take responsibility for self and the journey you choose for yourself before arrival on earth. I believe we basically plan our lifetime prior to birth. Each and every lifetime is for balancing to reach perfection, once balanced further lifetimes are not needed.

Love your parents, you chose them.

It's time to drop the pendulums, dowsing and muscle testing aids. Have faith that you as an evolved soul don't need them, they can misdirect you if your vibration is not attuned to high levels. Work for positive purity in all directions of your life, to allow your connection to the quantum level.

There is no going back, life is a constant move forward, or it should be.

Treat your body temple well, you have to live in it for a long time. You will never be able to love another until you love yourself. So, expand, come out of your body to know there is more to you, the place where your soul lives, the place where all is recorded for past lives and this one, your energy field.

Expand to enter new dimensional fields of magnificent feelings of love, colours you have never imagined, music, purity of thought, joy, bliss and happiness.

Index

accidents, 252–4, 256–63
adrenals, 82–3, 275
animals, 32, 37, 103, 171
    assisting humans, 180, 183, 184–5, 199–200
    death and injury, 95–6, 166, 180–4
    healing, 3, 180, 185–7, 194–9, 201–2, 209–10
    health, 187–8
ankles, 64, 85
arthritic extremities, 275–6

back pain, 23, 278–9
bacteria, 52, 60, 94, 115, 165, 168–9, 177
balance system, 80
bladder, 60, 61, 83, 84, 193, 280
bowel, 63, 177, 197–8, 275, 283
brain, 17, 43–4, 47–9
breasts, 53–4
Breath of Life technique, 27, 29, 53, 120–1, 138, 280
bronchioles, 81, 248

cancer and carcinoma, 46, 54, 99, 100, 108, 109, 160–1, 243
caster oil, 4, 158, 192, 268, 283
cataracts, 49, 50
Cauda Equina Syndrome, 280–1
children and babies, 7, 44, 65, 115, 123, 129, 130–5, 136–9, 153
colon, 62–3, 83, 186, 192, 198, 284

death desire, 108–9
deep vein thrombosis (DVT), 254–5
dimensional journey, 232–51
Divine Love, 14–15, 39, 44, 46, 97, 106, 111, 138, 219, 228, 237–8,
    247, 248
duodenal, 82, 275

E.coli, 170–1
ears, 65, 286
Einstein, Albert, 216–20, 224, 251, 292
elbows, 85
electromagnetic fields (EMF), 98, 114, 141–2, 150–6, 240, 241
electromagnetic hypersensitivity (EHS), 142–3
emotional problems, 69–88
Epsom salt baths, 64, 158, 192, 255, 275, 276, 283
exercise, 277–80
eyes, 49–50

fear, 2, 9, 24, 27, 36, 37, 45, 72–3, 77, 83, 85, 103, 141, 197–8,
    243, 253
feet, 286
food, 270–3

gallbladder, 16, 58–9, 60, 81–2, 84, 149, 172, 276
gallstones, 58, 149

hands, 85, 286
heart, 54–5, 81, 112, 135–6, 198
heart generator, 112, 135–6, 233, 236–7, 246, 248
hemorrhoids, 63
hips, 83–4, 262, 263
human energy field, 12, 19–20, 28, 30, 31, 42, 48, 49, 70, 78, 105–7,
    109–10, 183, 233, 237
  information stored, 118–19
  negativity, 28, 46, 113–18, 137–8, 140–1, 238, 239, 240–1, 245–6
  positive, 109–11, 119–21, 238, 246, 251

immune molecule, 46–7, 80, 156–7
immune system, 46–7
indigo children, 133–5
intestines, 57, 59, 82, 83, 84

kidney stones, 60, 270
kidneys, 60–1, 82–3, 286
knees, 63, 64, 85, 99, 100, 172

legs, 64, 254, 255, 263, 280
liver, 30, 35–6, 55–8, 60, 81, 82, 83, 84, 148, 158, 164, 167, 172, 175,
    254, 256, 262, 283
love, 72, 73, 97, 138, 289. see also Divine Love; unconditional love
lumbar, 84, 280
lungs, 52–3, 81, 84, 107–9, 157, 191, 192, 248, 255
lymphatics, 51–2, 81, 84, 191, 292

methicillin-resistant staphylococcus aureus (MRSA), 165, 168–70
milk thistle, 35–6, 158, 283
mind methods, 225–32
mobile phones, 46, 47–8, 114, 142, 152–7, 159, 166, 176, 241–2
mouth, 52, 188, 286
multi-dimensional reality, 234–7

narcolepsy, 99
neck, 64, 84
necrotising fasciitis, 169

obesity, 273–5
olive leaf oil extract, 282

pancreas, 60, 82, 84, 275
parasites, 56–7, 157, 164–5, 167, 175, 188, 189, 272, 273
pelvis, 83–4, 194, 195, 263
pituitary gland, 44–6, 80, 108, 191, 193, 262
poisoning, 30, 31, 52, 56, 114, 157, 158–9, 187, 189–94, 208
pregnancy, 122–9, 176–8, 252–3
prostate malfunction, 61–2, 83

reproductive system, 61–2, 83, 155

sacrum, 84–5
schizencephaly, 130–3
shoulders, 85
sinuses (nose), 50–1, 80, 286
skin, 66–7
spine, 64, 65–6, 84, 85, 263, 278, 279, 281
spleen, 60, 82, 84, 275
stomach, 59–60, 82
superstring theory, 234–5, 239

teeth, 80, 85–6, 196
thoracic, 84
throat, 51
thyroid, 39–40, 51, 80–1
tongue, 80
tumours, 9, 10, 48

unconditional love, 31–2, 44, 75, 77, 137, 199–200, 246

vibrational healing, 38, 144, 163, 183, 200, 287
vinegar, 158, 192, 255, 271, 275, 276–7, 283
viruses, 53, 56, 57, 96, 125, 157, 165, 167, 168, 191–2, 262

water, 269–70
worms, 56–7, 59, 164–8, 172–5, 177–8, 188–9
wrists, 85

• • • •

"Robyn, if it wasn't for the success of your loving work, I would now be in a wheelchair. You gave me back my quality of life, the ability to walk straight and tall, and be free of pain." — Janet, U.K.

"I was preparing to take my own life because of my suffering that no doctor or alternative practitioner could diagnose. You found it and eradicated it. I'm now perfectly well thanks to your method." — Nicky, Australia.

"I find it so interesting that my family and friends have actually seen my ailing body become well again. Yet, when I explain how you achieved this through telephone calls, from across the world, they just do not get it."
— Kate, U.K.

"You are probably the most amazing woman living on the planet today. Thanks for your dedication and bravery to show and prove your wellness approach. I celebrate every day the energetic life you gave me back. From the depth of my heart, thank you Robyn." — Liz, U.K.

"I was taught to go to the doctor if my body was troubled. Well I did, and became progressively worse, caught up in a merry go round of handfuls of pills, most added from the initial one or two, to cope with the side effects. Thank God my angels directed me to you, my liver and spine are now completely well; you did it all without pills, by phone. You are amazing."
— Gary, U.S.A.

"I was given an operation on my spine, which was totally unnecessary. You found the real reason why my spine was in such agony and healed it. Bless you Robyn." — Sandy, U.K.

• • • •